The International Libr

FATHERS OR SONS?

Founded by C. K. Ogden

The International Library of Psychology

PSYCHOANALYSIS
In 28 Volumes

FATHERS OR SONS?

A Study in Social Psychology

PRYNCE HOPKINS

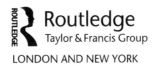
Routledge
Taylor & Francis Group
LONDON AND NEW YORK

First published in 1927
by Routledge, Trench, Trubner & Co., Ltd.
2 Park Square, Milton Park, Abingdon, Oxfordshire OX14 4RN
711 Third Avenue, New York, NY 10017

First issued in paperback 2014

Routledge is an imprint of the Taylor and Francis Group, an informa business

British Library Cataloguing in Publication Data
A CIP catalogue record for this book
is available from the British Library

Fathers Or Sons?
ISBN 0415-21094-1
Psychoanalysis: 28 Volumes
ISBN 0415-21132-8
The International Library of Psychology: 204 Volumes
ISBN 0415-19132-7

ISBN 13: 978-1-138-87560-9 (pbk)
ISBN 13: 978-0-415-21094-2 (hbk)

TO

J. C. FLÜGEL

IN APPRECIATION OF WHAT I OWE
TO HIS LECTURES AND FRIENDLY
INTEREST.

CONTENTS

PART I

CONTRA-FATHER MOTIVES

PART II

PRO-FATHER MOTIVES

GENERAL INTRODUCTION

It is necessary to say just a few words as to (1) what this work undertakes to prove, (2) how far the work has been done by previous writers, and (3) upon what hypothesis it chiefly rests.

(1) The present thesis takes as accepted the main body of psycho-analytic doctrine. I am aware that many of Freud's views are the subject of controversy ; I will, however, assume their validity. The essential argument of my thesis is that *attitudes which had their origin in the infantile relationship of father-son are often the true cause of the adult's orientation toward particular social movements.* In other words :

(a) The reasons given out by adherents of various social movements as sufficient grounds why they support, and why others should support, these movements, are often rationalizations of deeper-lying motives, which these adherents cannot acknowledge to themselves. It should, though, be needless to say that only the more extreme cases are to be regarded as necessarily, in Freud's sense, sexual.

(b) Among such unacknowledged motives are many derived from the feelings of the male infant towards his father or father-substitutes.

(2) *Previous studies have been made in this same field.*
The most considerable expositions along lines parallel to those we shall undertake are, (a) Freud's chapters on " Religious Practices " and on " ' Civilized ' Sexual Morality " in Volume II, and on " War " in Volume IV of his *Collected Papers ;* (b) Alexander Kolnai's *Psycho-Analysis and Sociology ;* (c) Dr Jones' introductory

chapters concerning " War " in his *Essays in Applied Psycho-Analysis* ; (d) J. C. Flügel's articles on the " International Language Movement ", in the *International Journal of Psychoanalysis*, and (e) the series of lectures given before Leplay House Sociological Trust by members of the British Psychoanalytical Society and published under the editorship of Dr Ernest Jones, as *Social Aspects of Psycho-Analysis*.

There have also been a large number of shorter contributions appearing from time to time in the various psycho-analytic journals, and of which the titles will be found in the various footnotes hereto.

(3) *Large portions of the present thesis rest upon what Freud calls the Œdipus complex.* As is well known, that theory assumes that a child normally loves best the parent of the opposite sex and is jealous of the parent of its own sex.[1]

The milder forms of such rivalry are easily observed. I have seen it in my small son, who, when less than a year old, used to become very irritated when his mother kissed me in his presence. Again, we had visiting us, last March, a three-and-a-half-year-old niece. One morning as I was leaving the house I pulled my wife into a room to kiss her good-bye, and, in fun, shut the door after us. Immediately the little niece, for whom we stood as parental surrogates, burst into tears.

In young children we may hear death wishes expressed

---

[1] " If anyone appears to be without jealousy 'we may be sure it is really there, but repressed ' and consequently plays all the greater part in his unconscious mental life. Jealousy is not necessarily ' derived from the actual situation ' at the time, but it is a left-over feeling which originated in the childhood ' family complex '." Freud (S.), " Certain Neurotic Mechanisms in Jealousy ", *International Journal of Psychoanalysis*, vol. IV, part I, p. 1.

" Of the infantile jealousies the most important . . . is the resentment felt by a boy towards his father when the latter disturbs, as he necessarily must, his enjoyment of his mother's exclusive affection.

" This feeling is the deepest source of the old world conflict between the younger and older generations, the favourite theme of so many poets and writers, the control motive of most mythologies and religions." Jones (E.), " A Psycho-Analytic Study of Hamlet ", in his *Essays in Applied Psycho-Analysis* (London, 1923), p. 16.

against the parent of like sex.[1] And they similarly find expression through his playing.[2] Mythology and folk lore also afford much correlative evidence in this field. There a constant theme, as in the myth of Œdipus, " is the success of a young hero displacing a rival father ".[3] Here, however, we enter controversial ground. The school represented by Elliot Smith have collected an amount of evidence for the hypothesis of the migration of culture (mummification with peculiar incisions, pyramids, the swastika, terraced agriculture, etc.) which cannot be lightly dismissed.

We should naturally expect, therefore, in sociology, too, to find the sons becoming heroes of revolutionary forces to oppose the conservative fathers. Ernest Jones, commenting on the opposition of sons to their fathers, which is due to the latter's superior rights over the mother, says this

" varies with—among other factors—the extent to which the aroused feelings have been repressed. . . . To this source many social revolutionaries—perhaps all—owe the original impetus of their rebelliousness against authority, as can often be plainly traced—for instance, with Shelley and Mirabeau."[4]

I have given so much space to the discussion of the Œdipus complex because its existence is less readily recognized than the existence of feelings friendly to the father. These latter, indeed, scarcely required to be commented upon at present.

Besides, many actions which pass current as being due

[1] von Hug-Hellmuth (H.), " On the Technique of Child Analysis ", *Int. Jour. of Psycho-Analysis* (London, 1921), vol. II, p. 295.
[2] Frau Klein has found that the play of young children is the most useful material obtainable for analysing them. In analyses described by her in lectures before the Psycho-Analytic Association in London during June and July, 1925, there appeared most convincing evidences of the Œdipus complex in each case recounted.
[3] Jones (E.), " Psycho-Analytic Study of Hamlet ", *Essays in Applied Psycho-Analysis*, pp. 73-4. See on this subject, Rank (Otto), *Der Mythus der Geburt des Helden*, 1909.
[4] Jones (E.), *Essays in Applied Psycho-Analysis*, p. 49. He refers to Wittels, *Tragische Motiv*, 1913, p. 153.

to love of the father are themselves more accurately described as reaction formations against repressed father-hatred. But enough of this topic.

Let me forestall an objection which may be made to the materials which I have selected to illustrate the points of my thesis. It will be said that the quotations I have given are extreme selections, and do not fairly represent the main body of adherents to the movements in question.

It is true that the selection has been of this kind, but I made it so deliberately, casting aside my earlier notes. The reader must bear in mind that it is not part of the purpose of this book to weigh the validity or social usefulness of the movements herein discussed. It is not a thesis in sociology, but in pathological psychology. As such it is much more aided by the review of arguments which have been pushed to the point of absurdity, than of those which would make the reader exclaim, " But this argument is just a legitimate deduction from facts ".

When an argument is stated with moderation and good judgment the skeleton of personal complexes which may be contained therein is hidden from view. But we may find another writer stating the case extravagantly. It is still the same point, but the rationalization has now worn thin, and the bones of the skeleton are laid bare for the psychologist to see.

I clearly recognize that the material presented in this thesis is not all of equal value. It falls into three types, which may be classed according to relative merit as follows :

1. Evidence of hitherto unobserved facts.

2. Application to the phenomena under discussion of evidence from other authorities, when the matter treated by them is so akin to our own that the jump is a very small one.

3. Arguments from analogy. Recognizing that these amount to little more than suggestions, I have en-

deavoured either to eliminate these or to express them very cautiously.

Finally, let me call attention to the synopsis of this book, which occupies its last ten pages. Some readers may prefer to glance at it first, the better to orientate themselves through the body of the work.

PART I
CONTRA-FATHER MOTIVES

PART I

CHAPTER I

THE RESCUE PHANTASY

INTRODUCTORY REMARKS

A CONDENSED statement of the *rescue phantasy* has been given by Flügel, much as follows : Thought of sexual relations between his parents is, because of jealousy and because of repressed incest wishes, distasteful to a child. So the son likes to imagine that his mother enters into such relations only because forced to by his father. Next, he dreams of " rescuing " her from such attentions. But since the idea of fighting his father is itself unwelcome to consciousness, the boy's phantasy disguises itself in legends like those of Andromeda or of St. George, in which a beautiful maiden (the boy's mother) is delivered by a young hero from a tyrant giant or monster. The same phantasy appears in the dream of delivering

" a small or helpless race or nation from the domination of a larger . . . or again by the struggle for the liberation of an oppressed section of the community from the tyranny of a ruling class ".[1]

This mania to save is commonly the motive for charitable work among the downtrodden. It must certainly have a place very often in the desire to save youths from

[1] *vide* Flügel (J. C.), *Psycho-Analytic Study of the Family* (London, 1924), pp. 108-9.

3

exploitation by corporations, which, by their wealth, their power, etc., recall the childish concepts of the father.

" The idea of rescue has a further symbolic meaning, which may be present to the Unconscious. To rescue means to save from death, i.e. to present with life, and thus comes to be equated with the notion of begetting or bringing into life. In this way the rescue of the mother may signify to the unconscious a begetting, i.e. a process of cohabitation with her. As a further determinant there is sometimes to be found an obscure notion of self begetting —the creating of oneself without the co-operation of the parent of one's own sex, all obligation to and connection with this parent being thus repudiated ".[1]

With regard to the rescue phantasy, I may mention an analysand of my own whom I shall call Gould. During the analysis he recollected at least one occasion when, as a child of six or so, he had pleaded with his drunken father not to strike his mother, who had crawled under the bed. The attitude of championing someone remained with him, although his father died soon after this time, and although Gould himself became estranged from his mother. At first, his little sister took the mother's place as someone to be protected ; and after her, a few other women came in for a brief share. But a strong homo-sexual tendency on which I shall comment presently seemed to block the development of all these affairs, and assisted in the substitution of various *groups* of people, or even *abstract* conceptions as the objects to be rescued. Thus he became the champion of various causes and left-wing movements, which he wished to rescue from the stern father-like government, from the war-drunk bourgeoisie, etc.

It may be objected that Gould's case was highly exceptional, inasmuch as most children do not have drunken brutal fathers. But it should be remembered that, given only a sufficiently strong motive for degrading

[1] Flügel (J. C.), *Psycho-Analytic Study of the Family* (London, 1924), pp. 108-9,

and hating the father, then what actual provocation reality fails to supply, is quite easily conjured up by a child's jealous fancy. So that, all in all,

"Saving phantasies, where that is to be saved from the 'wicked father' varies from a given person (e.g. Shelley's first wife) to the whole of mankind (democratic reform, etc.) are thus extremely common ".[1]

Occasionally, says Freud, dreams and daydreams show us in the act of rescuing some *father* figure. For instance, the patient dreams that he stops the runaway horses of a carriage in which the king is driving, and so saves the latter's life. But the analysis of such phantasies shows them to be only superficially acts of kindness to the father ; the carriage itself is usually a mother symbol, and the runaway action of the horses which the son so bravely stops represents parental coitus.

To this may be added the tendency, which Freud has already appreciated, of being " quits " with the father by saving his life ; the father now " owes " his life to his son, just as the latter " owes " his to the father.[2]

ECONOMICO POLITICAL TYPE OF MOVEMENTS

It is under the above title that I shall discuss socialism and allied movements. Quite a striking example of the identification of the king with the father and of the country with the mother is found in recent anti-Royalist utterances of Blasco Ibanez. This novelist has always been a romantic figure, espousing minority causes, fighting duels, etc.

[1] Jones (E.), " The God Complex ", in *Internationale Zeitschrift fur Psychoanalyse*, 1913, Bd. I, p. 313. Republished in his *Essays in Applied Psycho-Analysis*, (London, 1923), p. 224.

[2] " Freud pointed out that the tendency to rescue the father is chiefly the expression of an impulse of defiance on the son's part." Abraham (Karl), " Rescue and Murder of the Father in Neurotic Phantasies ", *Inter. Journ. of Psa.*, London, 1922, vol. III., part IV., pp. 267-8. See also p. 470.

Now, having written a book on "Alphonso XIII Unmasked ", he cries :

> " My country is like a lady of mediaeval romance imprisoned in a dark tower. Every man, in every country, owes it to the spirit of human freedom to liberate her ".[1]

But we shall see that the complexes which motivate individuals may motivate great masses.

Socialism

There exists a world-wide movement which is antagonistic to all such father-surrogates as kings, potentates, and ruling or possessing classes. (In the family circle the father is the wealth possessor.) This movement, socialism, champions the poor and dispossessed—those who are not masters but drudges, spending their lives serving and bearing children, and who so far resemble the mother. I suggest that thus through socialism the rescue motive finds considerable expression, even if special circumstances have determined that a Lord Shaftesbury[2] or a Tolstoy loving to rescue humanity should yet oppose the socialist method.

This great movement owes its present form largely to one outstanding figure—Karl Marx. And the chief representative of Marx in England was the late H. M. Hyndman.

It bears on my suggestion that the rescue motive is present in socialism, that Marx all his life was a romantic person (of somewhat the type of Ibanez). Well endowed intellectually, he was still more pronouncedly a man of strong emotions. He scorned the prosaic career which his father had planned for him, and spent his time at the University in writing poetry and in getting into and out of scrapes. He began early to interest himself in philosophical and economic move-

---

[1] Ibanez, Blasco ; as quoted by Slocombe (Geo.), in London *Daily Herald*, Oct. 18th, 1924.
[2] See quotation on pp. 18 and 19, below.

ments, and in championing the common people, with intent to rescue them from these father-figures of capitalist and kaiser. Various traits in common of Marx and Hyndman illustrate the fact that we tend to take as our leaders those whose complexes are similar to our own (whence we see the importance of learning the characteristics of these pioneers). Certainly Hyndman shared his master's romantic temperament. Bernard Shaw told him once,

" The truth is that you are an economic revolutionary on a mediaeval basis of pure chivalry—Bayard educated by Marx ".[1]

My hypothesis that the socialistic appeal takes root in tender feelings toward the mother, the first woman and first love object in every man's life, receives corroboration from an interesting detail in the history of socialist and communist experiments. For this we need not go earlier than the time of the Protestant Reformation, or revolt against the papal father. This period was the precursor to a great outburst of cults which advocated that property should be shared by all alike as it was by the early Christians.[2]

Radicalism and Morals

The detail to which I refer is the curious fact that innovations in marriage, also—in that sacrament whereby the father has exclusive claims on the mother—appeared among many of these sects. The best known is that of the Oneida community in New York State. After a time the Oneida colonists gave up their sexual peculiarities, yielding to public pressure. Some fifty years ago, though they had thrived they also gave up the communal form of property ownership, and were content to become a joint stock company, which still continues.

[1] Shaw (G. B.), in appendix to Hyndman (R. T.), *Last Days of H. M. Hyndman*, p. 289.
In a private conversation to which I shall allude, Mr. Shaw several times mentioned to me this romantic strain in Hyndman.
[2] See Brown (Bishop Montgomery), *Communism and Christianism*.

Frequently it happens that economically revolutionary movements are accompanied by a readjustment of ancestor-made, tradition-bound, barriers between the sexes. This takes sometimes the form of a looseness of such barriers, sometimes of so rigid an insistence upon them that one suspects herein an over-compensation has taken place.[1]

The intuitive perception of this fact, made keener by existence of like libidinous tendencies in oneself which one seeks to project on to others, and when coupled with bitter hostility against the sons, causes the father-minded newspapers to place the stigma of " free love " upon so many socialistic experiments. For example, the American Press were almost a unit in referring to the Brook Farm experiment in co-operative housekeeping (in that day a radical departure) as a free-love colony, although no shred of evidence of this was ever offered. Those who took part in it have this slander whispered about them to this day. More fresh in the public memory is the preposterous story about the " nationalization of women " by the Bolshevics. To be sure we do find among the utterances of Lenin this :

" At the very next concert meeting before an audience of thousands of people, there will be arranged on the platform a general kissing. A cadet lady lecturer will kiss Breshkovskaya. The latter will kiss the former minister Tseretelli, and a grateful people will thus learn the meaning of republican equality, liberty, and fraternity ".[2]

Between the father-admiring conservative and the son-admiring socialist, there is much bitter argument on the questions of sex and morality. The rebel sons say that the vice of prostitution results from the contrast between destitution and luxury. The fathers claim that it is due to a decline, for which the sons are respon-

---

[1] Although we must allow for the additional fact that the general propertylessness otherwise of the working-men may well make them the more ready to maintain a property attitude towards their wives.
[2] Lenin (N.), *Will the Bolshevics Be Able to Maintain Power ?* p. 67.

sible, in religion and in respect for authoritative (father-revering) moral standards.

To this last, the sons counter with the charge that it is precisely "upper class" (father identified) society which is most corrupt. Witness the following comment in the *New Leader* upon a recent famous scandal :

> " I know a good many socialists, and a few communists, but I doubt if among the whole pack of working people who count as socialists or communists you would find . . . that one man, in hopes of getting a ' step up ' allows his wife to give herself to the boss, or that the boss proposes such a bargain, or that the woman is to ' pay the price ". For that kind of mutual arrangement one must rout among the classes who are born to live at ease. You remember the story of the ' Diamond Necklace ' ? . . . the French Revolution followed close upon its shame, and the Society in which that drama was enacted, did not retain their enviable lot."[1]

Indeed, reverence for the fathers is said to have become impossible and to be in need of replacement by reverence for the new brotherhood. In Professor Karl Pearson's words :

> " It is because the old bases of religion and morality have become impossible to the present, that socialism—which gives us a rational motive for conduct, which demands from each individual service to Society and reverence to Society incorporated in the *State*—is destined to play such a large part in the reshaping of human institutions. Socialism . . . accepts no divine revelation as a basis of conduct ; it asserts the human origin, the plastic and developmental character, of morals."[2]

HUMANITARIAN TYPE OF MOVEMENTS

Now which particular one of its many possible forms will be assumed by the Rescue Phantasy, will, in each

[1] Nevinson (H. W.), " Our Heaven-sent Rulers," *New Leader*, London, March 27th, 1925.

[2] Pearson (Karl), *Ethics of Freethought* (London, 1888), p. 321.

instance, depend partly on what surrogates and symbols chance presents to the individual as suitable substitutes for the actual parent. We may be moved to rescue " fair humanity " from the brutality of war, but the rescue motive may in other cases actually oppose pacifists or other humanitarians.

Pacifism

For instance—as Jones has so beautifully described in his paper on " The Island of Ireland "[1]—one's native land may stand for either of the parents according to circumstances. More often it represents the mother. Witness our term " the mother country ". In such cases we have the explanation of the violent emotions stirred by the prospect of a foreign invasion, since the unconscious conceives of it in terms of a violation of the mother.

The enemy then comes in for all the infantile hostile feelings originally directed against the father. Moreover, these become in a degree fixated, and long outlast the period of actual hostilities. Thus, to most people in the allied countries, a German is still a hated father-surrogate.

When one's country, considered as the motherland, is substituted for the flesh and blood mother, then the rescue phantasy fires youth to rise in her defence against her enemies and detractors. The violation-phobia then is transferred from mother to motherland.[2]

In evidence of what is here asserted, let me call attention to the frequent use of an argument which confuses

---

[1] Jones (E.), *Essays in Applied Psycho-Analysis*, London, 1923.
[2] " We tend to regard our native land as a great mother who brings into being, nourishes, protects and cherishes her sons and daughters and inspires them with respect and love for herself and her traditions, customs, beliefs, and institutions, in return for which her children are prepared to work and fight for her . . . a good deal of the horror and disgust which is inspired by the idea of an invasion of one's native land by a hostile army is due to the unconscious tendency to regard such an invasion as a desecration and violation of the mother." Flügel (J. C.), *Psycho-Analytic Study of the Family* (London, 1924), p. 126.

pacifism, i.e. unwillingness to take part in the indiscriminately murderous mass-actions of one huge army against another such army, with the more extreme doctrine of complete non-resistance. The person (Hudson Maxim) using this argument in the question below—the stock question that was asked of all consciencious objectors in England—has been impelled to speak as though the invasion of the country were precisely like, or necessarily involved, the rape of the mother :

> " If, when this country is invaded, some militant scoundrel, forcing his way into your home, should lay the hand of violent lust on trembling wife or daughter, would you observe the pacifist policy of non-resistance, or would you kill him ? "[1]

Furthermore, one sometimes gets from the pens of writers whom one could never in the world accuse of sympathy with psycho-analysis, such flashes of insight as this :

> " So it [patriotism] is apt to act in the name of ' my country, right or wrong ', even if it means no more than Mr Chesterton's ' my mother, drunk or sober '."[2]

" But what," some writer may here object, " of those who conceive of their country not as a motherland but as a fatherland ? "

It is true that some so conceive of it ; and certain aspects of it, such as the *state* or the *government*, seem always to be thought of as Father. But that the implications so far as they concern the Œdipus complex remain much the same, I believe I have sufficiently indicated in the introductory remarks to this chapter, under the topic of *rescuing the father*.

Charitable Work

We have described how a child creates phantasies in which a hero (representing himself) rescues someone in

---

[1] Maxim (H.), *Defenceless America*, p. 305.
[2] *The World To-Morrow*, New York, February, 1924.

distress (the mother) from some wicked oppressor (the father). As we noted, the distressed object is often found in actual life in the person of some social unfortunate. Or animals and the helpless in general are associated to the mother, and so arouse the rescue phantasy. Thus :

> " Lord Shaftesbury, the seventh Earl . . . was in conflict with a tyrannical forbidding father, and the subject of his mother's neglect. The headmaster of the school to which he was early sent, was, according to all accounts, inhuman and brutal . . . There was, says one of his biographers, neither joy in going back to school, nor joy in coming home, where he was often left with insufficient food. It is easy to see the narcissistic projection in this Champion of Children, the Chairman of the Ragged Union, the reformer of asylums . . . There was another determinent . . . The sole person who seems to have bestowed any love on this unfortunate son of an earl was his mother's old maid. Until the day of his death Lord Shaftesbury wore a watch which this maid had left him in her will. His love for this woman of inferior station finds an expression in adult life in his efforts to amend the lot of the oppressed, the lowly, the humble, but he does not throw in his lot with them, he remains always faithful to his rôle of protector, of master ; nor apparently could his complexes allow him to regard an independent working-class with complacency—as you probably know he was the opponent of the education acts."[1]

It seems reasonable to presume that the mechanism which was responsible for bringing Lord Shaftesbury into charitable work must be operative in others also. The rescue phantasy would thus be indicated as an important source of such work in general.

RELIGIO-THERAPEUTIC TYPE OF MOVEMENTS

In the discussion on which we shall now enter, reference will be made so frequently to religious concepts and

---

[1] Eder (Dr M. D.), " Psycho-Analysis in Politics." See *Social Aspects of Psycho-Analysis*, edited by Jones (E.), (London, 1924), pp. 150-1.

authority, that we shall do well at this point to reinforce what has already been said with regard to their paternal origins. Thus, Freud tells us :

" Psycho-analytic investigation of the individual teaches with special emphasis that God is in every case modelled after the father and that our personal relation to God is dependent upon our relation to our physical father, fluctuating and changing with him, and that God at bottom is nothing but an exalted father."[1]

Dr Eder adds :

" Voltaire said that man had fashioned God in his own image ; it would be nearer to the mark to say, in the image of his father, i.e. of the ideal which is built up in the earliest years of childhood."[2]

On the genesis of the gods out of mortal clay, moreover, light is shed by such ancient customs as that of paying religious homage to kings (fathers of the tribe) during their lives. That hero worship was often literally the deification process in action is indicated by such sayings as that of Pythagoras :

" Reverence great heroes, and do them the rites that are due."[3]

[1] " Here also, as in the case of totemism, psycho-analysis advises us to believe the faithful, who call God father just as they called the totem their ancestor. If psycho-analysis deserves any consideration at all, then the share of father in idea of God must be very important, quite aside from all the other origins and meanings of God upon which psycho-analysis can throw no light." Freud (S.), *Totem and Taboo* (Transl. Brill, London), p. 244.
[2] Eder (M. D.), " Psycho-Analysis in Politics," in *Social Aspects of Psycho-Analysis* (Ed. by E. Jones, London, 1924), p. 134.
[3] *The Golden Words*, as quoted by Harrison (F.), *New Calendar*, London, 1923.
Says also Flügel : " The study of religion shows that the conceptions which religion has formed as to the nature and working of the Universe have arisen as products of the human emotions, having no necessary counterparts in the real world ; much the same indeed in this respect as the inventions of the fairy stories and imaginative games of childhood, of the day-dreams, romances and novels of a later age. In adult life such phantasies must either be abandoned or, if indulged in, recognized for what they are—productions of the mind which, apart from objective evidence, have no valid claim upon reality." Flügel (J. C.), *Psycho-Analytic Study of the Family* (London, 1923), p. 155.

That the origins of religious belief were largely phallic, has been long emphasized by various writers,[1] and is assimilated by Jones to psycho-analytic principles,[2] with especial animadversions on such topics as baptism[3] and sacrifice.[4] These must not be taken as justifying that crude type of rationalism which asserts that there is " nothing in " religious dogmas. The view-point is rather that there is a great deal " in " them, only not what we hitherto supposed. The dogmas represent real truths, but the truths concern not objective reality, but the believer himself. Indeed, a vague perception of this fact and an attempt to compromise with it, leads the proponents of various decaying creeds to place upon them sundry new interpretations more harmonious with modern science,

[1] See Moses (J.), *Some Pathological Aspects of Religions*, Clark University Press, U.S.A.

[2] " When the facts of Eastern phallic religions began to reach Europe in the nineteenth century, they seemed so incredible that they had at all costs to be re-interpreted into harmless terms, and the view, still prevalent, was adopted that the worship had nothing to do with the phallus as such, but was really directed towards the abstract idea of the divine creative power, which we personify, as the Creator, and for which the phallus was a ' symbol ' appropriate to simple minds. Reflection shows that the abstract idea in question must itself have been derived from the concrete idea symbolized by the phallic image."
Jones (E.), *The Theory of Symbolism. British Journal of Psychology*, vol. IX. Republished in his *Papers on Psycho-Analysis* (London, 1923), pp. 198-9.

[3] " Probably the simplest and most accurate expression for the psychological meaning of baptism, as perhaps for that of any religious rite, is ' purification through re-birth '. The earthly incestuous libido, which is now known to be the deepest source of the sense of sin in general, is overcome and purified in a homeopathic manner by passing through a symbolic act of heavenly incest." Jones (E.), " The Symbolic Significance of Salt," published in *Imago*, 1912, ed. 1, pp. 361 and 454. Republished in his *Essays in Applied Psycho-Analysis* (1923), p. 163.

[4] " The meaning of ' sacrifice' has been investigated by means of the psycho-analytic method by Freud. According to him, the . . . belief that mankind is to be saved from its sins through the sacrifice of Jesus Christ on the Cross, represents an elaboration of the primitive totemistic system. The essence of this system he sees in an attempt to allay the sense of guilt arising from the Œdipus complex." Jones (E.), " A Psycho-Analytic Study of the Holy Ghost." In his *Essays in Applied Psycho-Analysis* (1923), pp. 415-6,

or making them appear even to have forestalled the discoveries of science.[1]

The religious movements which will come within the purview of this thesis are those in which the healing or hardening of the body or " soul " of the believer is thought to be achieved through faith or special cultish practices doubtfully related to reality. Naturally, these movements are not on the best terms with scientific medicine.

It happens that a doctor is peculiarly liable to become a substitute for the father. He is the one outsider consulted by the family on the most serious crises ; he knows even more than the real father, and, especially about forbidden topics ; he is depended upon to take charge on important occasions ; etc.[2] So a father he becomes to the unconscious.

[1] A familiar example of this is the attempt by Gladstone in his famous controversy with Huxley to maintain that the biblical six-day creation story forestalled the scientific account of evolution, and was consistent with it if for " day ", one read " epoch ". (Unfortunately, as Huxley was able to show, the order of creation in Genesis is not identical with that postulated by Science).

Another example is afforded by Yogi apologists such as Sir J. G. Woodroffe (pseud. Arthur Avalon) in his *The Six Chakras and the Serpent Power* (London, 1919), who endeavours to show that the Chakras, or hypothetical centres which Yoga exercises are intended successively to " awaken ", correspond with the sinuses in the spinal column whence (the anatomy of a later day has shown) important groups of nerves leave the spinal column to control the legs, the internal organs, the arms, etc.

The first of these examples my readers would find too hackneyed a theme, were I to expand upon it. But I may be permitted to remark upon the second example, that the six or seven centres to be awakened in succession, are so regularly parallelled in other religions by seven virtues or seven stages in development, that one inclines to believe that these represent some imperfectly visioned subjective phenomena, e.g. perhaps the successive stages of libido-development.

[2] " The displacement on to medical advisers and attendants of feelings originally directed to parents, has frequently been recognized. . . . It is more particularly the attribute of benevolent omniscience that is liable to be transferred. Three factors contribute especially to this result. (1) The physicians ' knowledge on matters of the highest interest and importance, about which others are relatively ignorant (particularly perhaps ' medical matters ' in the sexual sense of that euphemism) ; (2) the fact that the situations in which his assistance is called in, for the most part urgently demand some kind of action which he alone can perform ; the sense of helplessness which others feel in these situations being similar in many respects to that frequently

Quimby and his Successors

When, therefore, the doctors come in for both the attributes of wickedness and father-likeness as we shall find they do from believers in faith cure, those who are treated by them, the women at any rate, will tend to be regarded as mothers to be rescued.

Thus P. P. Quimby, whom we shall come to know very intimately in these pages as the true founder of Christian Science and of New Thought, speaks of himself as a Moses come to lead the people out of

> " the sea of blood or blind beliefs into which the physicians have misled them."

Also we shall find him eager to save the " spirit " (generally pictured as feminine in works of art) from the semen-like thoughts of evil-minded doctors ; again a kind of rescue phantasy. And in at least one other place I have found him equating mind with matter, soil and earth (mother-symbols in mythology and in dreams) which he would apparently like to defend from being impregnated :

> " Disease is the disturbance of the mind or spiritual matter . . . mind is disturbed like the soil of the earth ready to receive the seed."[1]

The rescue motive is likewise apparent in Ralph Waldo Trine, when he hopes by means of his New Thought teachings to save Mother from the dreadful misadventure of poisoning her child (the rescuer's self). He avers :

experienced in earlier years when, as children, we were dependent upon the efforts of our parents in many of the important affairs of life ; (3) the fact that this sense of helplessness and the general attitude of suggestibility are still further increased in the case of the patient by the general regression to a relatively childish state of mind which illness so frequently brings in its train." Flügel (J. C.), *Psycho-Analytic Study of the Family* (London, 1924), pp. 120-1.

[1] Quimby (P. P.), see Dresser (H. W.), *Quimby Manuscripts* (London), p. 180,

" We have seen several well-authenticated cases of the following nature :

" A mother has been dominated for a few moments by an intense passion of anger, and the child at her breast has died within an hour's time, so poisoned had become the mother's milk."[1]

It is not surprising to find that such a believer in thought power as is Mrs Eddy countenances the doctrine of pre-natal influence. This she does in a sentence which emphasizes her elsewhere-expressed position that the physical factor in marriage is unimportant (child's feigning of contemptuous indifference to copulation between the parents) :

" The offspring of heavenly-minded parents inherit more intellect, better-balanced minds, and sounder constitutions."[2]

(By heavenly-mindedness, presumably is meant freedom from worldly or carnal thoughts, such as passion between father and mother.)

Pre-natal influence is endorsed by Coué " in sober truth, if a woman a few weeks after conception " suitably impresses her mind.[3]

A pointed case

An especially enlightening case of rescue phantasy is that of a young man who has turned away from religion because assent to it as expounded by the Church Elders (fathers) would have involved acquiescence in the damnation of a woman he revered. The autobiography

---

[1] Trine (R. W.), *In Tune with the Infinite* (London, 1923), p. 32. By the way, why does he describe the cases as " well authenticated " if he himself saw them ?

[2] Eddy (Mrs M.A.M.B.G.P.), *Science and Health*, p. 16.

[3] Leon (Mme Emile), *Thoughts and Precepts of Coué, circa* p. 38. A further development of the child's unwillingness to admit that the beloved parent has physical sexual relations with the other and hated parent, is to be found, as it appears to me, in the dislike of admitting the existence of a physical world at all, which rings through the whole Berkeley-Quimby-Eddy school of metaphysics. As Jones somewhere remarks, our word *material* is derived from the Latin *mater*, mother.

of this man[1] begins with a description of his elaborate dogmatic schooling in the healing sect of Seventh Day Adventists. When he graduated from their theological seminary, his professor said of him that if all copies of the New Testament were lost, Nash would be able to replace them from memory.

Starting fervently, then, upon his career as pastor, he became acquainted with an exceedingly good old lady, whose work had been to restore ex-criminals to honesty and self respect. When this lady died, Nash's ecclesiastical superior demanded that he should assent to the judgment that, since she hadn't been converted to Adventism, she must be eternally damned. The effect was to make him reject the whole body of Adventist teachings.

The point I wish to make is, that Nash immediately flew to the extreme of opposition against every ideal of life connected with his early beliefs. He became an atheist, and a tramp and an outcast as well, and so remained for a long period. In order to effect the rescue of a motherly woman symbolically from the hell preached by the church elders, his life should give the lie to their cruel religion.

Let us sum up, now, this chapter. We have seen the rescue phantasy illustrated most poignantly in the cases of Ibanez and Shaftesbury. But the movements of Socialism and Communism seem, like their founder, Marx, to have been motivated largely by the rescue motive. It is obviously present in humanitarianism, in the soldier's desire to fight for his mother country, in such cult-founders as Quimby, Mrs Eddy and Coué, and in the type of hostility to religion for a while represented by Nash.

---

[1] Nash, *The Golden Rule in Business.*

CHAPTER II

THE FATHER AS AGGRESSOR, OPPRESSOR, CRIMINAL, ETC.

INTRODUCTORY REMARKS

THE father is the successful rival of the son for possession of the mother. Another important aspect in which he appears is as the impersonalization of power. This aspect, as Freud says, originally was

" embodied by the child in the conception of the father ; and the desire for power is the desire to rival and displace the father."[1]

We have mentioned the interesting way in which the infant creates phantasies upon the basis of the situation between his parents, imagining that his mother is the unassenting victim of assault by his father, and picturing himself as the hero destined to rescue her.

But Freud has shown that this primitive jealousy does not stop short of definite accusations against the father. By the carelessness of parents, who generally are ignorant of such susceptibilities, and of the extent of interest and of comprehension in infants, coitus is often performed in the same room in which baby has his own cot. The little fellow becomes both curious and alarmed at the sound of heavy breathing. He is only too ready to believe that the father is making some sort of attack on his beloved mother. His vanity leads him fondly to imagine that she loves only himself, hence must be struggling against this assault. The father, therefore, is all the more a villain ; he is, indeed, the prototype in

[1] Freud (S.), *Totem and Tabu* (Transl. Brill), p. 143.

the likeness of which are constructed all future villains,
rapers, robbers, marauders, violators, etc.

The attitude of the child who is rankling with what
he considers the injustice of his father's rule in the
household may become ingrained. The naughty boy
develops then into the chronic rebel.

In the degree that real arbitrariness or injustice by
his father increases the alienation from him of his son,
the latter is thrown more and more into the arms of his
mother. His love becomes concentrated the more upon
her. Or it may be that some other figure in the family
receives this benefit, but one who is, in reality, a mother-
substitute, e.g. an aunt.

The father has the right to interfere in all the family
plans. His word is generally the final one. He is,
therefore, the prototype of autocrat, absolutist, king,
monarch or tyrant ; and he stands for the principles of
authority and power.

Inasmuch as the legislation of any earthly father is
often unwise, and as still more of his conduct is un-
agreeable to his children's wishes, so that they become
rebels, he is forced into the position of the suppressor of
rebellion. In him the children find the model for the
legislator, the lawyer, the judge, the conservative, hence,
further, for the legislating or ruling class, the legal
profession, and the conservative parties.

Of individuals who by their profession come in naturally for the feelings meant for the father, there are
several. Little children are often heard at first to call
all men " daddy ". Only slightly more restricted is the
usage in some savage tribes, where one calls every male
of the older generation of the tribe, Father. The
civilized child is soon corrected in this use of the term.
But inadvertently he still retains a feeling of men being
all somewhat of a class with his father. More especially
does he manifest this strongly with regard to uncles and
elder brothers, who, like the father, wield a certain
authority over him.

Let me, however, caution the reader against assuming son-hatred and father-hatred to be necessarily different entities. Resentment against the father sometimes shows itself in measures which imply a repudiation of the position of the father, or a reversal of it relatively to the son.[1]

ECONOMICO-POLITICAL TYPE

In the cases now to be considered, what is denied is the authority of the father. Who is he, ask the sons, that no other voice than his may make itself heard? Or, veiling this repressed thought, and substituting a surrogate for the father, who are these lawyers and justices that they should bring injunctions against peaceful picketing? Who are our constabulary that they should take a hand against us strikers? etc.

Dr M. D. Eder has observed that the identification of oneself with other children of the family against the father is the origin of the sentiment from which later arise the slogans: " Liberté, Egalité, Fraternité ", and " workers of the world unite ", together with the concept of the class war.[2]

[1] e.g. Suppose A to be the father and B the son. When B grows up and marries, and has a son of his own, C, there are many things which make him tend to identify C unacknowledgedly with A. For C has come between B and the woman B now loves (B's wife) as, a generation earlier, A stood between B and the woman he loved at that time, namely B's mother. In the present position of having C in his power, B reacts as though it were A whom he had in his power.

Thus the alternate generations come to be equated, and, *pari passu*, grandfather and grandson come to league themselves against the father.

[2] " Identification with other children of the family or little friends can become in adult life identification with the people . . . ' justice for me ' becomes ' justice for all ', ' equal rights for all ', and we get the famous slogan ' workers of the world unite ', ' you have a world to gain, you have nothing to lose but your chains '. It is the effect arising from this hostility of the children towards the father (the possessor) that gives force to the abstract conception of the class war. Then arises another father, another God: ' The voice of the people is the voice of God '—an instance of what Ferenczi calls the infantile happy condition of omnipotence." Eder (M. D.), " Psycho-Analysis in Politics," in *Social Aspects of Psycho-Analysis*, ed. by E. Jones (London, 1924).

Flügel points out that the primitive tendency of human beings is, when faced with any difficulty, to blame fellow beings instead of seeking some scientific explanation and way out. In complicated modern life, the differences in fortune between men are peculiarly obvious, and the processes of wealth-creation difficult to observe. So nature is regarded as a beneficient all-providing mother, only thwarted by wicked father figures.[1]

We shall see this tendency cropping up as we proceed to various discussions below under the headings of Karl Marx, Hyndman, Anti-Socialist Utterances, Superficial Aspects of Democracy, Shielding from Competition and Anarchism.

Karl Marx

There is surely reason to believe that such hostility as this theory calls for did exist between Karl Marx and his father. We know that in spite of brilliant intellectual endowments, Karl failed miserably at school and at college. Though naturally studious, Karl " spent his time at Bonn in youthful escapades and follies " so that his disappointed father transferred him to the University

[1] " We have been accustomed all through our history (human and prehuman) to compete with other beings. . . . The struggle for existence has indeed fostered this tendency, eliminating those whose ability to assert themselves against competitors was insufficient. This being the case, we still tend in the face of any difficulty or disaster to turn in anger against our fellow men rather than to seek for the explanation and correction of our troubles in terms of natural science.

" Owing to the complexity of social and economic factors . . . the difference in fortune between man and man becomes exceedingly conspicuous, while the fundamental facts connected with the production of food and other necessaries are rendered difficult of observation. Under these circumstances it becomes only too easy to assume (with the imperialistically inclined) that all shortages of the necessaries of life are due to the competition of other nations, peoples or races, or (with the socialistically inclined) to the injustice and tyranny of certain classes. Here, again, *parental complexes* are often at work. Nature being regarded, as before, as the beneficient mother who means well by her children, while the human enemies or oppressors are regarded by a process of displacement from those originally directed to the hated father." Flügel (J. C.), " Biological Basis of Sexual Repression," *Brit. Journal of Medical Psychology*, vol. I, p. 257.

at Berlin. Here, again, however, he gave himself to every pursuit except that which his father desired, and failed to pass his examination.

> " His father became vexed . . . and many angry letters Marx senior wrote to his son reproaching him for his conduct."

At last the boy

> " in distress and disgrace . . . came home to his parents' house . . . His father, unhappy at his son's conduct, was lying in bed in the throes of an incurable disease."

In short, the son had succeeded in hastening, by unfilial conduct, his father's death.

Consciously, of course, both men tender a display of affection toward each other. "But the trouble ", continues the biographer I am quoting,

> " lay in their generation, and in the chasm of intellectual [sic !] differences that had sprung up. His father sank in his illness and died . . . leaving his son to tread revolutionary paths . . . which would have caused the old lawyer many heartaches had he lived to see it."[1]

As is constantly shown in the analysis of " political complexes ", the state, which inherits that position of authority over the individual first occupied by the father, inherits with it the father's place in the individual's affections. If, in the case we are considering, the state came in at the start for none too happy a heritage, it made its identification with the father still

---

[1] " At Berlin, Karl . . . hated legal study, but delighted in wandering through the realm of philosophy, metaphysical speculation and historical and literary romanticism. But all this led to no practical result. Marx studied, and read and dreamed. He sketched out great plans of future success as poet, as author, as dramatist, and indeed scribbled volumes of poetry, novels, plays and essays, but could not bring himself to pass the necessary college examinations and earn the acadamic degrees that would open up a practical career. His father became vexed at his unworldly son dreaming and bemusing his time away. . . . In distress and disgrace he came home to his parents' house. His father, unhappy at his son's conduct, was lying in bed in the throes of an incurable disease." Cooke (A. E.), *Socialism of Karl Marx* (Glasgow, 1918), p. 3.

stronger in Marx's imagination, by arbitrary displays of force. First, the official Prussian attitude towards Jews (even Christianized ones) made him resign all hopes of a career as a scholar. Next, when he turned to publishing a (radical) paper, this paper was suppressed. Experiences with foreign governments presently convinced him that they, too, were of one class.

In view of the close affinity between the governing class and the wealthy, Marx's condemnation of autocracy as one of the objectional points in capitalism was to be expected,[1] even were it not preconditioned by the fact that in the family group the father is both capitalist and governor in one.

> "His father, Heinrich Marx, was a lawyer of Jewish birth, a descendant of a long line of Jewish Rabbis, and an official of the Prussian Government, as well as a justice of the peace . . . He was a loyal conservative, and an upholder of the Prussian State . . . He represented a type . . . breathing kindness, culture, and broadmindedness in his intellectual side and in his home circle, but outside of that, in the harsh world of every-day existence, was dominated by the 'practical side' of things, the 'hard cash' basis. Really a liberal by virtue of thought and reading, but a tory because of the worldly advantages accruing therefrom."[2]

The factor, therefore, of a rebellious early relationship toward, at any rate, his father, is a fairly safe matter for presumption. It is to be placed alongside of doctrinaire and persecution mania tendencies in contributing to his hatred of bourgeois control of governments. Marx's father was a bourgeois.

---

[1] *Idem.*

[2] Cooke (A. E.), *Socialism of Karl Marx* (Glasgow, 1918), p. 1. Toward his mother, apparently, Karl's attitude was more loving than it was toward his father. Yet of her, even, we are told that " she asserted no intellectual influence over him." Cooke (A. E.), *Socialism of Karl Marx*, p. 3.

And later, " Karl's mother . . . oft was almost heartbroken at her rebel son, defying the forces of governments, and giving forth to the world the revolutionary message of socialism ". Cooke (A. E.), *Socialism of Karl Marx*, p. 3.

Marx's literary tastes were in keeping with the dictates of the Œdipus complex. In poetry :

" He liked in particular Walt Whitman, the Prophet of Democracy, and was specially fond of ' Pioneers, O Pioneers '."[1]

In short, quite aside from the logic by which he justified his actions, Marx was obviously acting in accord with his rebel temperament, for which socialism was the most important of several possible channels of expression.

A somewhat different part of Marx's character may be responsible for certain errors of judgment which have been a weapon in the hands of his opponents, namely :

" As to his judgment of men, it is enough to say that he was too tolerant of his estimates on one side and too bitter on the other."[2]

One suspects that this lack of balance was most probably due to an unsatisfactory relationship with the first man to come into his life, the relationship which was to become the archtype of all future ones with men, namely with that of his father. This may have been due to a reaction against homo-sexual love for the father —a subject of which we shall treat in Chapter IV. Otherwise we can best attribute it to the Œdipus Complex.

Marx's declamations against the capitalist system itself, and still more against the bourgeoisie as a class, declamations full of fire because they picture that class as a sort of evil demon father deliberately conspiring against the happiness of the masses—all these strike one as remarkably like his merely personal attacks. They might all be but variations on his denunciations of his personal opponents.

Herweg, Hertzen, and Bakunin, all were denounced

---

[1] Salter (F. R.), *Karl Marx and Modern Socialism* (London, 1921), pp. 6-7.
[2] Hyndman (H. M.), *Record of an Adventurous Life* (London, 1911), p. 275.

by him as tools of reactionary governments. In the case of the last named, the charge was twice repeated by Marx after he had substantial proof of its falsity.[1]

Naturally the persons most likely to be thought of as punishing—and later, as persecuting—him, will be those that lend themselves to association to the persons who punished him in childhood, i.e. especially father-surrogates. But now I will leave for a time these deductions concerning Marx, in order to tell the reader about someone concerning whom I have personal knowledge.

Every juvenile judge or truant officer knows that although a small boy whom he arrests is the leader of a gang and the most mischievous element in it, the boy's parents will almost invariably be certain that their darling was led astray by some older companion. The following is an instance. The mother of Kenyon, a neurotic, of whom frequent mention will be made in these pages, well illustrated this mechanism. As soon as she noted that her son was manifesting certain leanings toward radicalism, she at once decided that this must be due to the malign influence of a young assistant in his business who sometimes expressed mild right-wing socialistic views. Chiefly on this account[2] the mother

[1] " In 1848 he denounced Herweg as a reactionary tool, for no other reason apparently than that he appeared not to favour Herweg's proposal for raising a revolutionary legion to go out and fight.

" In Germany, Hertzen was accused in the same manner later, as was, of all people, Bakunin. In 1824 there appeared in the *Neue Rheinische Zeitung*, which Marx was then editing a report from Paris to the effect that George Sand . . . was in possession of proof that Bakunin was nothing less than a tool of the Russian Government.

" The infuriated anarchist at once wrote to George Sand demanding an explanation, whereupon it was discovered that she knew nothing about the matter. Marx apologised. . . . [But] the charge was repeated in 1850, again without the production of any proof, in the *Morning Advertiser*. . . .

" Yet once more, in 1862, the old accusation appeared . . . in the ' exile ' circles of London there was general agreement that it had been written by Marx." Salter (F. R.), *Karl Marx and Modern Socialism* (London, 1921), pp. 46-7.

[2] The young man's expressions did, it is true, draw upon the institution some scandal-mongering attention from the reactionary elements of a small town.

presented the young man with his expenses for a journey to the Orient. At twenty-eight, Kenyon pioneered in organizing the freer intellectual elements of the town into a Liberal Club, and thereafter he induced some of them to assist him in writing and distributing pacifist literature during the war, and for this he was arrested. The mother, on both these occasions, was convinced that her ewe lamb had been seduced by his wicked comrades, and later she found an opportunity of inflicting rather severe injury upon the estate of one of them.

We see this mechanism cropping up constantly in the sociological argument. The popularity or spread of any movement is accounted for by its opponents on the ground that innocent people in their childlike naïvete have been seduced by some wicked " professional "— or father. We are always hearing that revolutions and strikes are not due to anything whatever except the speeches (symbolic potency) of agitators. Regarding free trade, also,

" Those who hold this view have been led astray by the false teachings of professional economists."[1]

Returning now to Karl Marx, I will conclude my observations with a story Mr Bernard Shaw told me about him.[2]

" Marx ", said Mr Shaw, " was intensely jealous ! " and he went on to relate how the father of modern socialism came finally to break with his faithful follower, Hyndman. It seems that, about 1880, Hyndman wrote a short book on economics which, in effect, was a summary of the principles of socialism. But as Marx's name was anathema in England, Hyndman, in order that the book might be more generally read, referred to Marx only as " a well-known German economist ". For this

---

[1] Young (J. P.), *Protection and Progress* (Chicago, 1900), p. 11. Whether the writer prefers amateurism in economics, he leaves us to infer.

[2] In a private conversation, November 27th, 1924.

Marx broke with him, and, up to his death, a year later, never forgave him.

" Marx's wife, though ", Mr Shaw went on, " had a different explanation of the falling out. She said : ' One day Hyndman by mistake put on Marx's hat, and it fitted him so perfectly that he walked away with it ! ' "

As a ground for a quarrel between friends Mrs Marx's hypothesis is quite ludicrous. But it seems to me a very pretty illustration of psycho-analytic mechanisms, for that very reason. For who can fail to see the significance of this so symbolic episode between these two strangely egotistic men, the master so soon to die, and the pupil who, in England, was to succeed him ?

Mr J. C. Flügel tells me that he had once an analysand who was obsessed with the phantasy of grabbing the hat off a man on a passing 'bus ; and this on analysis proved to be a castration phantasy. So does Father Marx seem to have regarded Hyndman's running off with his hat ; that likewise was a gesture of castration.

Hyndman

I have related that the great representative of Marx in England was J. M. Hyndman. He, like William Morris[1] and so many other revolutionaries, sprang of conservative parents. Hyndman's father bequested £150,000 of his property away from his son to a religious foundation, and the son on his part reciprocated the paternal mistrust. In the private conversation already alluded to, Mr Shaw said that during all the years of his and Hyndman's intimacy, the latter " never once referred to his father, mother or childhood. Apparently he wanted to imply that he had never been anything but a full-grown man of the world ".

" Self created out of nothing, like God ? " I asked. Mr Shaw laughed and conceded that this fitted the case.

---

[1] The conditions of his family surrounded him with conservatism. He was born of affluent parents whose wealth increased during his childhood and youth. Stickney (G.), *William Morris*, p. 3.

Already he had written, in his introduction to Rosalind Hyndman's biography of her husband's *Last Days*,

" Apparently he did not care a rap for his own father."[1]

Certainly in his autobiography *Hyndman* is at no pains to conceal a thorough-going disapproval of his father's ideals, and to question even his general business competence.

The question of family prosperity is, of course, peculiarly one which in later life is likely to be projected into the field of political economy. The father is the first known monopolist of (family) property. Between him and the children, who hold their few meagre possessions only at his pleasure, yawns a gulf. To-day, millions of persons are at once the employees of others, while at the same time through owning a few tools or property which they rent out, or a few shares in some joint stock company or co-operative society, they are small capitalists. Marx's prediction of a growth in a contrary direction has not been justified. So we arrive at this striking inference. That utter chasm which Marx projected into the future of public affairs lay really in the past and in his own relation to his father.

In our own day *Nicolæ Lenin*, although the modern world lay before his eyes, yet exaggeratedly stated that a condition of hard and fast division was present in it to-day :[2]

" ' The whole world,' said he, ' is divided into two camps. " We," the labouring class, and " they," the exploiters.'."[3]

Some anti-Socialist utterances

But that the rebellious-son spirit may align people against, instead of in favour of, socialism, is often

---

[1] Shaw (B.), in appendix to Hyndman (R.), *Last Days of H. M. Hyndman* (London, 1923), p. 268.

[2] See page 170 for an equally sweeping denial of any such division.

[3] Ulianov (V. ; Lenin, N.), *Will the Bolsheviks Maintain Power ?* (London, 1922), p. 85.

apparent. For instance, the internationalism of Marx, which we have seen to have been a revolt against states as fathers, is looked upon by others as being a slight to the mother-land. By these people Marx himself is regarded as the offending father. The fact of him being a German, of course, facilitates this attitude. And so socialism

> " Unfortunately—and this is by far the most serious aspect of the matter—is part of an international movement . . . Marx . . . used this international movement for furthering German designs. Ever since his day German social democracy has dominated the international socialist movement . . . Our Socialists have to-day placed themselves again under the same domination by affiliating themselves to the Hamburg International, and subordinating the party to the control of that body in international affairs."[1]

But although Marx's international attitude, so generally shared by his followers, was anti-state, there is much in his philosophy which is distinctly favourable to the state —a new state, more democratically governed, but still a state. The father is to be overthrown, but in order that the son may step into his place. In view of this tendency, and regarding the socialist state as all the more a father because it is to be the all-owner, and all-employer, we can understand how some rebellious sons will not welcome, but rather oppose it. This spirit is heard in the alarmed cry of Professor Flint :

> " Contemporary socialism desires to serve itself heir to the absolution of past ages. Its spirit is identical with that of all absolutisms. It seeks to deify itself, and means to brook no resistance to its will."[2]

Hilaire Belloc, similarly, fears that if the community were converted to socialism at all it would surely be

---

[1] Northumberland in introduction to Mallock (H. H.), *Democracy* (London, 1924), p. xi.
[2] Flint (Prof. J.), *Socialism*, p. 227.

converted to the most oppressive form of it.   But he consoles himself that a

> " force making against the establishment of socialism . . .
> [is that] you will never get the run of men and women con-
> tented to live their whole lives entirely under orders . . .
> Of liberty . . . under socialism [a man or woman] would
> have none.   He would have to do what he was told by his
> taskmasters . . . Not a part of his life, nor so many hours
> a day, but the whole of life would be subject to orders given
> by others."[1]

Similarly the Rt. Hon. Asquith :

> " The great loss balancing all apparent gains of a re-
> construction of society upon what were socialistic lines,
> would be that liberty would be slowly but surely starved . . .
> and that we should have the most startling despotism that
> the world had ever seen."[2]

The individualist arguments find their own extreme expression in the anarchist assertion that to have any father (State) at all is misery for the sons (labour—the numerous and dependent) and that when the sons are strong enough it will be all up with him :

> " The state rests on the slavery of labour.   If labour
> becomes free, the state is lost."[3]

Superficial Aspects of Democracy

One of the strongest motives towards economic radicalism is the desire to do away with distinction of classes—there shall no longer be some fathers and others sons, but all shall be brothers.

In Russia to-day, so I am told by Paul Birnhoff, friend and biographer of Tolstoy, this vision has largely become a reality, except among a few officials carried over from the old régime and among the new profiteering

---

[1] Belloc (Hilaire), *Economics for Helen* (N.Y., 1924), p. 124.
[2] Asquith (Rt. Hon., M.P.), quoted in *Anti-Socialist Speakers' Handbook* (London, 1911), p. 11.
[3] Quoted by Sprading (Chas.), *Liberty and the Great Libertarians*.
Los Angeles.

class which has sprung up since the reintroduction of capitalism. As an evidence of the change of spirit, he cites the fact that practically no interest is taken by men as to how they *dress*.

In the city of New York this democratic sentiment regarding outer appearance is travestied in regard to men's headgear. On the first of July, every man is expected to wear a flat straw hat of standard pattern, and to continue until the first of September, when he is to discard it in favour of a bowler or felt hat. This rule is so strictly obeyed that the view of a New York crowd say, from a 'bus at the noon hour when all business houses are emptying, is an unforgettable sight—a sea of thousands of exactly similar heads. Moreover, the fervour of sartorial egalitarianism in New York surpasses that in Moscow in that compliance is more or less compulsory ; a bowler hat worn on July 2nd, or a straw hat on September 2nd is likely to be crushed over the wearer's eyes. However, all this is excess of standardization, of course, and not true democracy, nor an expression of working-class sentiment.

Corresponding to this, a kind of mental egalitarianism exists in certain quarters which shows itself in suspicion of experts in any field.[1]

Moreover, the comparatively good system of common schools endeavours to raise the stock of information of all persons to a common level. Lest some should rise above this level many states have legislated as to what facts may be discussed by teachers. The recent Tennessee trial of a schoolmaster for teaching evolution has given publicity to the intellectual egalitarianism of the fundamentalists, who would standarize biological theory on the basis of such facts as were known to Moses. There must be no intellectual giants (fathers) competing with us.

---

[1] However, a general title to be heard respectfully on any subject from medicine to social theory is granted to outstanding business men,

Shielding from Competition

A tendency to shield the individual from too much competition in the economic field is present in socialism. A tendency to shelter various *businesses* from the rough world manifests itself in *protectionism*. The very name, " infant industries ", is used in my own country in every political campaign to enlist the chivalrous instincts of the voter in defence of such concerns (although actually they are enormous and flourishing) as the sugar " trust " and the steel " trust " against the terror of foreign competition. I submit that the word *infant* gives us the clue to the situation ; repressed memories of our own infancy, when we clung to our mother, are stirred up, and we are asked to identify ourselves with the mewling sugar trust. The intuitive naming of foreign competition an " ogre " or " bogey " by opponents of protection is further evidence for us, since Freud has pointed out that ogres and bogeys are simply father-images.

In the writings of an English protectionist I find a different though yet more preposterous argument which seems to mean that from practically all rivalry of the father, it is always the duty of the mother to protect her little boy(s) :

> " From . . . practically all foreign competition it is always the duty of the state to afford its citizens' industries shelter."[1]

In active politics as much as in the economic theorizing which we have just discussed, the attitude of the child towards his father will affect that of the man toward what has taken the father's place—for instance, toward the party temporarily in power.

The child may, as Flügel says,[2] react in either of two opposite ways to the managerial tendencies, especially when excessive, of his parent. The less wholesome way

---

[1] Williams (Ernest E.), *Case for Protection* (London, 1899), pp. 32-3.
[2] Flügel (J. C.), *The Psycho-Analytic Study of the Family* (London, 1923).

is that he may give in to them entirely, becoming meekly over-submissive. The more vigorous way is to develop a truculent spirit of independence. In this manner is generated that passionate championship of the principle of freedom, which appears in libertarianism of various types.

Anarchism

Generally the father-defying impulses tend to enlist one against, rather than on the side of, censoriousness and regulating. But, however impulsive such action may be in its real essence, it is generally rationalized in terms of some altruistic principle.

Wm. von Humbolt says that :

> " In proportion as each individual relies upon the helpful vigilence of the state, he learns to abandon to its responsibility the fate and well being of his fellow citizens. But the inevitable tendency of such abandonment is to deaden the living force of sympathy, and to render the natural impulse to mutual assistance inactive."

Max Stirner declares :

> " The state always has the sole purpose to limit, tame, subordinate, the individual, to make him subject of some generality or other."

Paine is of opinion that :

> " The trade of governing has always been monopolized by the most ignorant and most rascally individuals of mankind."

Shelley agrees with these views, and explains that of necessity :

> " Power, like a devastating pestilence,
> Pollutes what e'er it touches,"

The moral to be drawn from these beliefs for practical action is not far to seek. In the words of Dr Clifford :

" All our liberties are due to men who, when their conscience has compelled them, have broken the laws of the land."[1]

In like vein hear Emerson :

" It will never make any difference to a hero what the laws are."

Another writer declares :

" There is one thing in the world more wicked than the desire to command, and that is the will to obey."[2]

Against the autocratic assumption of domestic authority the son reacts in favour of more rights and privileges for the rest of the family. This may include a championing of his mother, or it may be purely a conspiracy of the younger members of the family against the older.

In political life, this spirit is the genesis of democracy.

Politics is the management of public affairs, and thus corresponds to functions in the original household which generally the father allocated to himself. To usurp them, therefore, puts the usurper in the father's place.

Naturally the hostility to the father is an important factor in every sort of political movement, since the persons who occupy office in the state become *ipso facto* father surrogates.

" Psycho-analytic work has shown that a ruler, whether king, emperor, president, or what not . . . tends to draw on to himself the ambivalent attitude characteristic of the son's feelings for the father . . . The most complete nonentity may, if only he finds himself in the special position of kingship, be regarded either as a model of all the virtues,

---

[1] Dr Clifford, quoted by Sprading (Chas. T.), " Laconics of Liberty " in his *Liberty and the Great Libertians* (Los Angeles, 1923), p. 34.

[2] See Sprading, *supra*, p. 34.

to whom deference is due, or as a heartless tyrant whom it would be a good act to hurl from his throne."[1]

An interesting confirmation of this was given by Sir Flinders Petrie in a lecture in which he mentioned that there was hardly a tomb of the Egyptian Pharoahs but had been opened within a few minutes of its sealing and the king torn to bits.

This hostility to rulers, going beyond the rational, interferes in various ways with sanity of political action. While in general it is anything but a conservative force, it can generally be so manipulated as to defeat any constructive revolutionary action. Thus, in most countries there exist two political parties which differ from each other in little more than name, both being supported by subscriptions from the same corporations. It is a constant complaint of the left wing parties that popular political interest stops short at the point of turning out the " ins " and replacing them by the " outs " from the other of the two parties mentioned. Afterward they turn out the second and let the first ones in again, *ad infinitum*, the whole being merely emotional unintelligent reaction. But this is what we have learned to expect where the turning-out impulse is based not on outward reality but on an inner complex, the original instigator and object of which was the individual's father.[2]

---

[1] Jones (E.), *A Psycho-Analytic Study of Hamlet*. First printed in the American Journal of Psychology, Jan. 1910. Reprinted in his *Essays in Applied Psycho-Analysis* (1923), pp. 67-8.

[2] " These conflicting relationships—tenderness, the wish to be like the father in every way ; and hostility, the wish to be rid of the father—exist side by side, just as we have seen the one tie, identification, spreading out and finding a number of partial substitutes. Thus the hostility may be felt by the child toward the father himself, and the tenderness towards an uncle, a teacher, the gardener, the dog, a collection of stamps or butterflies. The reversed case is also possible. . . .

" For this fission of affects the British Constitution provides admirably. I think it was Mr Zangwill who once said that the king can do no wrong and his ministers no right. That is to say that the ambivalency originally experienced towards the father is now split ; the sentiment of loyalty, etc., is now displaced on to the king, the hostility on to the king's ministers, or on to some of them, the Opposition, the Labour Party, etc. The President of a Republic such as the French, is in

With some, the protest against there being any superiors whatever assumes sweeping form :

" The great are only great because we are on our knees. Let us arise ! "

So says Max Stirner, who also declares :

" Individually free is he who is responsible to no man . . . This freedom of man is, in political liberalism, freedom from persons, from personal dominion, from the master. The securing of each individual person against another person, personal freedom."

Thomas Paine, religious heretic, humanist, and democrat, piles calumnies upon the origin of government :

" It is impossible that such governments as have hitherto existed in the world, could have commenced by any other means than a total violation of every principle, sacred and moral. The obscurity in which the origin of all the present governments is buried, implies the iniquity and disgrace with which they began."

Not only are governments and their officials assimilated to the father by dint of being in the seat of authority, but they revel in the employment of methods which remind the citizen of his parent. I refer here not only to the employment of coercive force against individuals and groups, but also to the delight in shrouding certain matters from the community with secrecy.

" At the back of secret diplomacy, trade secrets, and indeed the whole relationship of the official to the non-official, there rests this father-child affect."[1]

much the same case, but in the United States . . . the President comes in for the hostility reserved for the government in power . . . President Wilson . . . for a time . . . was the projected ego-ideal of a large mass of American mankind ; then came the surge of parricidal impulses and the President is hurled from power with every expression of ignominy." Eder (Dr M. D.), " Psycho-Analysis in Politics " in *Social Aspects of Psycho-Analysis*, ed. by E. Jones (London, 1924), pp. 138-41.

[1] Eder (Dr M. D.), " Psycho-Analysis in Politics " *Social Aspects of Psycho-Analysis*, ed. by E. Jones (London, 1924), p. 141.

Father reserves certain information (chiefly sexual) as not suited to the minds of the young. The latter must wait long before they are initiated and so made in this respect the equals of their parents.

HUMANITARIAN TYPE

An edifying study of the bearing upon a man's philosophy of his relationship with his father is found in the case of Jeremy Bentham, the founder of Utilitarianism and a noted democratic reformer and humanitarian. We shall also see a similar attitude working beneath the revolt of entire subject races against their masters and in international ill-feeling against a creditor nation.

Jeremy Bentham

Bentham senior seems not to have shown much sympathy toward his son, so that the latter's boyhood passed in a constant craving for happiness.[1] Jeremy reciprocated by so acting as to be a thorn in the flesh of his parent. Among other things he scouted the desire of Bentham senior to make of him a practical man of affairs, by becoming instead a speculative and social philosopher and social reformer. He relates :

> " While my father lived my conduct may indeed have sometimes been a cause of regret and dissatisfaction to him ; but on what ground ? My ' weakness and imprudence ' in keeping wrapt up in a napkin the talents which it had pleased God to confer on me—in rendering useless, as he averred, my powers of raising myself to the pinnacle of prosperity . . . He was continually telling me that everything was to

[1] " Bentham's father had . . . not the slightest comprehension of the delicacy and diffidence of his son's nature. He whose maturer and later life flowed in one stream of continued happiness—the most gay and joyous of men—had the recollection of his boyhood associated with many thoughts of a painful and gloomy character." Bowring (J.), *Works of Jeremy Bentham* (Edinburgh, 1843), vol x, p. 5.

be done by ' pushing ' ; but all his arguments failed to prevail on me to assume the requisite energy."[1]

He flouted his sire's sentiments,[2] made little good use of his time at college, and lampooned his father's profession (the law). Of his under-graduate days at Oxford he says :

> " We just went to the foolish lectures of our tutors to be taught something of logical jargon. I learnt nothing."[3]

His biographer quotes him to the effect

> " that the streets of Oxford were paved with perjury . . . After graduating he returned (at 16) to attend the lectures of Blackstone—and in due course to do his best, in his *Fragment on Government*, to demolish the lecturer. When he passed from the University to the Bar . . . he did his best to ' put to death ', and not without success, the cases which his anxious father had, as a solicitor, thrown in his way . . . If the reader will turn to the copious index to Bowring's edition of *Bentham's Works*, he will find under the heading ' Lawyers ' . . . :

" *Lawyers.*	Interest of, in the incogniscibility of the law.
,,	Mendacity, licence of.
,,	The only persons in whom ignorance of the law is not punished.
,,	Least of all men exposed to the operations of humanity.
,,	Opinion of, that cheap justice is bad, and dear justice good.
,,	Knowledge of, confined to the corrupt parts of human nature.
,,	Accessories to the crime they defend.
,,	Their interest in technical jargon.

---

[1] Bowring (J.), *ibid*, vol. x, p. 5.
[2] " Bentham's father . . . adopted for the family motto : *Tam bene quam benigne ;* and when Bentham was very young he was called on to translate the phrase . . . meant to convey a recondite meaning— *Tam bene*, read backwards was to designate *Bentham.* The lad neither valued the wit nor preserved the motto." Bowring (J.), *Works of Jeremy Bentham* (Edinb., 1843), vol. x, p. 5.
[3] Bowring (J.), *Works : Life of Bentham.*

" It had been the dearest ambition of Bentham's pushing
father to educate his own son to be a great lawyer . . .
The product was the most subversive critic that English
law and lawyers have ever had to encounter."[1]

Even after his father's death, Jeremy Bentham pursued
the latter's memory with unfavourable comments, and
justified this course by philosophic rationalizations :

" Bentham made, throughout his life, open war upon the
maxim *De mortuis nil nisi bonum* ; and as he frequently
spoke of his father in terms of disapprobation, he was in the
habit of justifying the course he pursued, by something like
the following reasoning :
" Why should a Latin or an English proverb screen an
ancestor from investigation ? The suppression of truth
may be as baneful as the utterance of untruth . . . Take
the case of flattery bestowed on dead tyrants. What does
it serve but to encourage a continuance or a repetition ? "[2]

It is in keeping with the principles elucidated by
psycho-analysis, that this unhappy child and *enfant
terrible* should become the apostle of hedonism, the man
who introduced into parliament the principle that the
ultimate happiness of the people should be the test of
rightness of every act, the champion of a widespread
suffrage, and, in general, of heretical and democratic
ideals.

I wish next to bring forward some considerations
regarding that humanitarian movement known as
pacifism. There is reason to believe that the childhood
impulse to defy the father as oppressor, often motivates
both those who espouse this movement and those who
oppose it.

As far as patriotism meant father-attachment, so far
may indifference or hostility to nationalism be an outgrowth of early repressed antagonism to the father.
Internationalism very often represents such a rejection

---

[1] MacCunn (John), *Six Radical Thinkers* (London, 1907), pp. 3 and 4.
[2] Bowring (J.), *Works of Jeremy Bentham* (Edinb., 1843), vol. x, p. 4.

of patriotic claims and, therefore, I maintain, of paternal ones.

But how can the defiance of the father lead in other instances to a more ardent patriotism? Chiefly, no doubt, by being projected on to other nations, not one's own. Let me illustrate.

Revolt of Subject Races

I have before me an essay upon The Rising Consciousness of Nationality, which forcibly illustrates the part played in this feeling by the Œdipus Complex. This essay refers back to the fulfilled prophecy made by the first British administrator in India, as to " the effect upon the character of a people of unqualified submission to an arbitrary foreign power."[1] The terms used repeat almost word for word those of J. C. Flügel when he is discussing psycho-analytically the dangers of similar submission of a child to its parents.

The article—whose author doubtless would have been horrified at the thought that he was giving evidence on behalf of applied psycho-analysis[2]—proceeds to describe what is clearly a collective castration complex :

"One of the chief complaints of the Indians to-day is that through the decades, they have been progressively emasculated, enfeebled in spirit and initiative impulse, and rendered incapable of doing anything but lean in a state of moral paralysis upon a protective paternalism."

It cannot be without significance that this writer chooses words like *emasculated* and *paternalism*. I myself, when in India, was struck by the fact that the most bitter opponents of the existing régime, when they had some reform to propose, would not say : Let *us* do it, but instead : Let *Government* (personified with a capital G) do it.

---

[1] The article appeared in the *Saturday Evening Post*, New York, Sept. 15th, 1923.
[2] The publication is perhaps the most reactionary weekly in the United States.

It is not only in India where he stands for the governing race that the Briton is a father figure. Throughout the East, Europeans—Britons and Americans especially— fit into this rôle. They are treated as lords. And this is natural, since they seem to possess all prestige, science, wealth and potency. But let us return to the news article.

In Hong Kong, the Chinese sons "may safely assume an attitude of indifference to British superiority" (a father attribute) and "are no longer respectful" (an attitude certainly first learnt toward the parents and especially the father).

The American in Japan meets "an attitude of self-confident arrogance" (over-compensation for tendency to be humble in presence of the father) "modified by an insistent enquiry as to Japanese rights of equality in spheres both social" (privileges with the mother) "and economic" (share in the family property) "among the great powers of the earth". (Great ones—fathers.)

"You get in Japan a rapidly developing Anglo-phobia" due to the policy of the British Admiralty (punitive power of the father). "You get also a deep resentment against the United States on account of an alleged colossal injustice" (the old family feud).

The next step is, of course, for the brothers to forget their mutual quarrels, in alliance against the old man :

"At the same time apparently open and above-board negotiations are in progress with the soviet authorities of Russia looking to the establishment of a Russo-Japanese *modus vivendi* on lines mutually beneficial."

although, since the article was published, events in Shanghai have interfered with this development by forcing Japan into the father rôles of employer and policeman.[1]

International Ill-feeling

Interesting in further respect of international relations is a remark which I hear made to the point of monotonous

[1] In making the above generalizations, I appreciate that the Far Eastern Question is complex. I would not be understood as trying to sum it all up in these few paragraphs.

repetition by my (American) compatriots in Europe. It is that " they all hate us over here ". The remark is usually accompanied with an air of bewilderment that it should be true, and of accusations of European ingratitude in view of our extensive charities and loans.

I suggest that the explanation is that precisely her financial favours have put the United States in a parental position. Her rôle of the world's banker arouses against her all the *anti*-father hatred which has always made the word money-lender odious. And that America is now so looked on, can be seen by glancing at dispatches in papers quite free from Jingoism ; as witness this reference in the *New Leader* to

> " Gigantic changes in the relations of America to Europe. Last week she settled Belgium's business. The epoch of sentiment towards that victim is over, and henceforth she will pay for the wrongs she suffered at the rate of £786,000 a year. The debt will run till 1987—if nothing happens in the meantime. When France and Italy are similarly brought to book, America will be the world's usurer."

And the bankers or usurers—are these not, as I have tried to show above, father-surrogates ?

Such are some of the ways in which hatred of the father tends to menace the peacefulness of international relations. But in other cases it leads some persons to combat these very tendencies to friction.

Thus the attempt of each nation to attain security by being better armed than all others and so frightening them off, as well as the actual endeavour to achieve idealistic aims by warlike means, have reminded some of Lowell's lines :

> " Attempt the Future's portal with the Past's blood-rusted key."[1]

Now, the lock and key have long been recognized as symbols, respectively, for the female and male genitals.

[1] Quoted by " X——", *Preparedness of America.*

The poet's verse symbolically portrays an act of sexual assault. The disparaging term *blood-rusted* carries with it implications of there having been a resistance (such as the boy's egotism makes him attribute to his mother when approached lustfully by his father, and as may be perhaps the result of chance observations connected with menstruation).

Let us now examine another pacifist utterance. Eden Philpotts, in his poem, *War*, after picturing the foulness (anal attribute) of war, says "to this the pomp and splendour" (regal or father-attributes) "of it comes". He is, therefore, debasing these paternal qualities. The next line is about "the burden of their country's yoke", that is, the distastefulness of obedience to the parents. The stanza closes with an emphasis on the doubtfulness of all things—the attitude experienced by children for probably the first time as a result of parental subterfuges when the child wishes to know about birth.[1]

Of European pacifists, the most famous was Leof Tolstoy. I have been unable to obtain anything directly about his relations to his father. It seems probable, however, that an Œdipus Complex existed in his case because, from all accounts,[2] Leof seems to have had a stronger transference toward his mother than would easily have brooked a rival :

"Though he could not remember his mother, Tolstoy tells us ' she appeared to me as a creature so elevated, pure and spiritual that often in the middle period of my life, during my struggles with overwhelming temptations, I prayed to her soul, begging her to aid me, and such prayer always helped me much.' "[3]

I have now to take up another complex mechanism

---

[1] Philpotts (Eden), " War ", quoted by Minermus in *Freethinker*, London, July, 1925.
[2] I refer particularly to verbal communications I had in August, 1925, with his biographer, Paul Birnkoff, in Geneva. Leof Tolstoy lost his father when Leof was a child.
[3] Maude (A.), *Leo Tolstoy* (Lond., 1918), p. 2.

resulting in pacifist sympathy. The reader will recall our remarks anent jealousy of existing or prospective other children giving rise to enthusiasm for the birth-control movement. It follows that if we come upon an argument *versus* nationalistic imperialism which is deduced from a fear of such imperialism interfering with birth control, we may suspect this to be really sprung from a fear that the imperialist father will insist on further child-bearing by the mother. Here is an example :

" Imperialism is a factor making for a large birth rate, e.g. imperialist propaganda for increase of population in France, legal restrictions on birth control propaganda in U.S.A., in Germany before the war, and by prohibition of public lectures by Mrs Sanger in Japan."

This opens up the topic of the close interconnection of militarism with capitalism, and consequently, of pacifism with socialism. As the socialist represents the father by dint of his wealth and consequent power and social position, so does the militarist by reason of embodying the idea of force.[1] The result is, that the rebel who sees his father in the capitalist, is predisposed also to see him in the militarist, and *vice versa.*

The pacifist, therefore, points out to the socialist that every war strengthens the position of the economic masters, by leaving the greater proportion of property in the hands of the few. The socialist, in his turn, dilates to the pacifist on munition interests and commercial rivalry for foreign markets as causes of militarism.

The genesis of the international spirit in the founder of socialism is superficially traceable in experiences of his young manhood :

" When Marx finally settled down in London in 1849 he had enjoyed the distinction of being expelled from three European countries . . .
" Marx, therefore, entered on his English period as an ' international man ' by necessity rather than choice."[2]

[1] We shall offer our readers proofs of this assertion in chapter III.
[2] Salter (F. R.), *Karl Marx and Modern Socialism* (London, 1921).

Sometimes the position of the conscientious objector involves the acme of resistance by the physically weaker yet unyielding party or child, against his powerful and infuriated father, in which if the little fellow has the requisite courage he may at length see his huge opponent retire angry and baffled. This can be illustrated from many an experience during the Great War. The one below, taken from a letter which one Ivan Sussoff wrote to his wife, describes a happening typical of many which occurred :

> "An officer . . . said, 'You must become soldiers' . . . 'We will force you to'. We answered, 'Force is with you . . .'
> "When they found that none of us would obey their orders, they commanded to turn the water on and put the fire hose against our faces. After being tortured like that for two hours, half dead we were dragged back to prison . . .
> "We refused to eat, and did not eat for eight days . . . They dragged me like an animal with rope round my neck. That peeled the skin off my neck . . . they threw me into an ice cold bath. I did not count how many times they beat me. Once in one of those ice-cold baths I fainted, and they took me out and tortured me again. They pulled the hair off my feet like feathers."

The book in which the above is found then continues :

> "A group of Molokans reached the jail. Their religion taught them that under no circumstances could they obey military orders. An officer was to them an officer, whether in a camp or in a prison. Because these men were foreigners . . . it was more of a temptation for low-grade guards to treat them brutally."[1]

Note the sentence, "an officer was to them an officer". Indeed, a father is always a father to the rebel son. The foreign immigrant in the United States is also, compared to the native inhabitants, peculiarly in the position of the unschooled and unskilful son to his educated father who knows how to do everything, has been longer in the world, owns property, etc.

[1] Thomas (Norman), *The Conscientious Objector* (New York), pp. 188-90

Another motive was given to the objector in the last war by the extent to which the governments carried their policy of allowing citizens no freedom of discussion of public affairs. In Chapter III below, under the caption of Political Movements, I claim to show that censorship, or the cutting off of the son's speech, is a symbolical castration by the father. Therefore, a defence against castration is what appears in the following as an argument against war :

> " Intolerance will continue after the cessation of hostilities to suppress those whose opinions are distasteful.
> " On the basis of the national hysteria and intolerance fomented by propaganda and persecution during the last war, Professor Chafee states that after the next war, critical thinking in this country will be practically impossible."[1]

RELIGIO-THERAPEUTIC TYPE

Upon the whole, those who are fundamentally hostile to the father will be hostile to those who worship his deified image in the skies. Just as[2] there have always been lovers of the father to whom it is inconceivable that any atheist can be a good man, so there have been persons who showed their hatred of the father by suspecting the motives of all who honour him. One is inclined to attribute some such repressed feeling to one who makes the sweeping generalization :

> " Morally the Christian is a bad mind because it has sought to place this submission to doctrine which it calls God, as a higher thing than individual development ; socially it is a bad mind, because it contributes nothing to the general good ; economically it is a bad mind, because its institutions exist by pauperage on society ; and politi-

[1] Chafee (Prof. Z.), *Propaganda and Conscription in the Next War*, New York, 1925 ; and a review of same by *Press Service of the Amercian Civil Liberties Union*. N.Y., May 13th, 1925.
[2] As we shall see in Part II, below.

cally it is the worst of minds, for whenever it had power it has sought to meddle with the simple procedure of existence, to impose its code of rules by bloodshed, and to attack in every way the effort of intellect to advance by its own private conviction."[1]

Indeed, the term Free Thought, which is used so generally as a synonym for Rationalism, has practically the same symbolic significations as one which we shall find in the term Free Speech. Thought and Speech are shown by Jones, in his " Psycho-Analytic Study of the Holy Ghost,"[2] to be in some cases potency symbols derived from associations with paternal flatus.

To *fertilize with an idea* is, thus, no arbitrary figure of speech ; and to declare oneself a *free-thinker*, or to uphold the rights of *free-thought*, is therefore to vaunt or to defend one's own potency as against the rivalrous father's.

Occasionally we shall find the feelings that arose out of antagonism to the father pulling on the side of religion instead of against it, but that will usually be in some new cult which has come out in rebellion against more established creeds, or else it will be because the antagonism to his father took the form of fear and submission rather than of a bolder attitude.

As regards newness, it happens that this designation applies to those cults I have in mind here to consider, which trace their origin to P. P. Quimby or Mrs Eddy, or belong to the New Thought school of which R. W. Trine is a representative.

---

[1] Lindsay (Norman), *Creative Effort*, as quoted by Yearsley (M. C.), in *Literary Guide*, Sept., 1925.

[2] Jones (E.), *Essays in Applied Psycho-Analysis* (London, 1923), p. 415 ff.
In another essay also he says : " Both the ideas of speech and of thinking are equivalent in the unconscious to that of passing flatus, which they frequently symbolise in consciousness." Jones (E.), " Hate and Anal. Erotism." *Int. Zeitschr. f. artl. Psychoanalyse*, Jour. I. Heft. 5. Republished in his *Papers on Psycho-Analysis*, 3rd ed., London, 1923.

P. P. Quimby

The movements to be discussed in this section of my thesis are largely developments of the theories and therapeutic methods of a New England physician, Phineas Parkhurst Quimby—not to trace them to the earlier sources, such as Berkeley, from whom Quimby got the philosophic seed of them. It was from Quimby that Mrs Eddy took over almost bodily the system which she capitalized under the name of Christian Science.[1] Now Quimby very interestingly equates thought with *seed* (semen). Using the ancient coitus symbol of *sowing*[2] (i.e. fertilizing the earth-mother), he gives us a passage in which a virgin spirit is described as having a live thing implanted in her by an evil agency unnamed ; i.e. the mother is raped. He says :

" Thought, like the seed, germinates and comes forth like the tree . . . Illustrations : a thought is sown in the mind while asleep or ignorant ; it grows and comes forth. The curiosity tastes ; it produces a strange sensation in the throat. The spirit enquires, the answer comes, bronchitis. The spirit is disturbed and tries to rid itself of its enemy. This disturbance is the effect called disease.

[1] " Quimby's writings were loaned to patients and followers who were especially interested, and after February, 1862, copies of his *Questions and Answers* were kept in circulation among patients. Mrs Eddy, then Mrs Patterson, had the full benefits of these exceptional opportunities. . . . Mr Dresser, who understood Quimby's ideas and methods particularly well, talked at length with her, and later loaned her Vol. I. of the manuscripts. . . . We learn from George Quimby, who, as his father's secretary was always present, that she talked at length with Dr Quimby, in his office, at the close of the silent sittings. She was present in the groups of interested listeners. ، . . She heard essays read and discussed.
" Submitting some of her first attempts at expressing the new ideas in her own way, she also had the benefit of Dr Quimby's criticism. Then too she had the opportunity to copy *Questions and Answers* on which she was later to base her teachings. We have direct testimony on all these points from those in direct association with Dr Quimby, and from those who knew Mrs Eddy when she was noting down remembered sayings and modifying manuscripts preparatory to teaching." Dresser (H. W.), *Quimby MSS.*, London, p. 12.
[2] Above, under head of " Rescuing the Mother," we quoted from Quimby that " mind is disturbed like the soil of the earth ready to receive the seed ".

" Now, if no name had been given or fears excited, the idea or tree would have died of itself."[1]

Mrs M. A. M. B. G. P. Eddy

Clues pointing to a similar unconscious dislike that the parents should have intercourse is revealed in several passages in Mrs Eddy's *Science and Health ;* as where she lays it down that :

" The formations of mortals must greatly improve to advance mankind. The scientific morals of marriage is spiritual unity. If the propagation of a higher human species is necessary to reach this goal, then its material conditions can only be permitted for the purpose of generating. The fœtus must be kept mentally pure and the gestation have the sanctity of virginity."[2]
" Mortals can never understand God's creation while believing that man is a creator. God's children already created will be cognised only as man finds the truth of being . . . No longer to marry nor to be ' given in marriage ' neither closes man's continuity nor his sense of increasing number in God's infinite plan."[3]

In the habit of submission to the father is laid the basis of that susceptibility to authoritatively given commands which has gone under the name of mesmerism and hypnotism. As is well known there are two methods of inducing the hypnotic state. One is by gentle soothing conversation, recalling, says Ferenczi, the influence of parental (and especially maternal) love. The other is through incisive commands, fear, etc., which Ferenczi likens to commands of the father.[4]

Now Quimby, before he developed the therapeutic

---

[1] Quimby (P. P.), see Dresser (H. W.), *Quimby MSS.*, London, p. 180.
[2] Eddy (Mrs M. A. M. B. G. P.), *Science and Health* (Boston, 1906), pp. 61-2.
[3] Eddy (Mrs M. A. M. B. G. P.), *Science and Health*, p. 60.
[4] Ferenczi, *Contributions to Psycho-Analysis*, transl. Jones, chap. II, pp. 57 ff.

ideas which were peculiar to him, was a noted mesmerist.[1]

He had, that is to say, an extraordinary power of calling up in persons their filial attitudes, whether of fear or of love. We shall therefore expect to find these attitudes cropping out among those who were later to become his cult followers.

The fact that Quimby rather than Mrs Eddy was the real source makes it more regular to treat of some of the Christian Science doctrines under the head of father-*son* antagonism. Moreover, Mrs Eddy herself seems to have experienced trouble in playing the ordinary feminine rôle. Her difficulty in finding marital happiness is testified to not only by the number of her husbands but by the cynical language in which, like St Paul, she speaks of marriage :

> " The time cometh of which Jesus spake when he declared that there should be no more marrying nor giving in marriage, but man would be as the angels. Then shall soul rejoice in its own, in which passion has no part. Then white-robed purity shall unite in one person masculine wisdom and feminine love, spiritual understanding and perpetual peace.
> " Until it is learned that God is the father of all, marriage will continue."[2]

Now psycho-analytic research has shown that relationship to one's mate is coloured by the relationship which existed to one's oppositely-sexed parent. Therefore one suspects that Mrs Eddy always found some difficulty in playing a normal feminine rôle, and that toward her stern and often harsh father Mary may well have manifested many of the feelings which are more natural for a

---

[1] " He met with a young man named Lucius Beirkmar over whom he had the most wonderful influence ; and it is not stating it too strongly to assert that with him he made some of the most astonishing exhibitions of mesmerism and clairvoyance that have been given in modern times." Quimby (G. A.), in *New England Magazine*, March, 1888, quoted by Dresser (A. G.), *Philosophy of P. P. Quimby*, p. 13.

[2] Eddy (Mrs M. A. M. B. G. P.), *Science and Health* (Boston, 1906), p. 64.

son than for a daughter to feel. In this case anything in the way of rescue of the father or of persons such as brothers who would be natural father surrogates, would appear to be covering devices to screen hostility, just as we saw was the case when a *son* dreams of rescuing them.

Whether by such a reaction-formation or through direct genuine attachment Mary seems, in fact, and at an early age, to have shown such concern about the souls of her brothers and sisters that on one occasion this worry brought upon her a serious fever :

> " From the earliest years she had been accustomed to listen to the theological discussions in which her father and his clerical friends took part. They were all strong Calvinists, believers in the doctrine of predestination. The little girl was greatly troubled by this doctrine. She was very much attached to her brothers and sisters, and . . . did not wish to be saved if they were to be numbered among those doomed to perpetual banishment from God's presence.
>
> " Mary Baker was much alarmed at the child's heretical views, and, hoping to win her from them, drew terrible pictures of the judgment day and eternal damnation. Mary's distress of mind at last brought on a fever, and the agonized father drove at a gallop for the doctor, thinking he was to lose his little girl body and soul. The family physician ordered complete rest and quiet, and left Mary in her mother's charge. As Mrs Baker bathed her little daughter's burning brow, she spoke to her of the great love of God, and told her to turn to Him in prayer, as she had been accustomed to do. It was Mary's first experience of spiritual healing."[1]

This incident has seemed to me worth quoting (in spite of some question as to whether the motives involved can properly come under the head of the present thesis) because of the light it seems to shed upon the genesis of the main Christian Science principle in the infant mind of the person who was to be its particular organiser. The fact that her mother was the one to exert such therapeutic power over her is additional reason for

[1] Ramsay (E. M.), *Christian Science* (Cambridge, 1924), pp. 8-9.

believing Mary to have been very homo-sexual. So also is the fact that she calls the deity " Father-Mother-God ", not merely Father.

If to the above we add the fact that a physician, as we have seen, is *par excellence* a father surrogate, it would have been strange had the coldness of the medical profession toward Christian Science not resurrected some very hostile feelings in its compiler.

Assuming this as so, one result of the admission must be to make us ascribe to a period a few years earlier at least than her writings the time when the future Mrs Eddy saw the medical fraternity as an enemy. In short, she must have seen them through Quimby's eyes. For her then strong transference toward Quimby, born of gratitude for the help and instruction he had given her, is witnessed by sonnets she soon afterwards wrote to him.[1]

Regarding Quimby, and not Mrs Eddy, as the source out of which came Christian Science (and, largely the New Thought movement as well), we are, as I have said, in a more logical position to speak of the evidence therein of *son* toward-father emotions. Quimby's own writings show a hostility to the profession of medicine ; this hostility he may well have bequeathed to his more famous patient, pupil and plagiarist.

It is difficult to obtain many significant facts about the infancy of Quimby. There is ground, however, to suppose that some accusations were levelled by him against his father for not having provided more abundantly the means whereby education would have been obtainable.[2] This, taken in conjunction with Quimby's extreme desire, on which we shall touch later, to reduce his therapy to a science, is reason from a psycho-analytic

---

[1] Dresser.
[2] " Owing to his father's scanty means and to the meagre chances for schooling, his opportunity for acquiring an education was limited. . . . He always regretted his lack of education." Quimby (G. A.), in *New England Magazine*, March, 1888. Quoted by Dresser (Anneita Gertrude), *Philosophy of P. P. Quimby* (Boston, 1895), pp. 11-12.

view-point for suspecting that his hostility to the parents was aroused by secretiveness on their part on the question, so intriguing to children, of where babies come from. Some question like this seems to have been so handled as to arouse in him a controversial tendency as well as an early aversion to accepting facts on mere hear-say (as though he resented some early deception practised on him by someone in whom he trusted).[1]

The infancy of Mrs Eddy was marked by neurotic illness for which physicians were unable to give her any relief—a fact which may well have excited her resentment against them as fathers who would not perform the function expected of them.[2]

Neither was the most recent famous advocate of mental therapy, Emile Coué, a robust child.[3] We may presume that, as in the case of Mrs Eddy, his experience with physicians was at least not of a kind to give him much confidence in them.

Often the father attitude spreads (via the individual doctor) till it takes as object the medical profession as a whole. Its conservatism, its reputation for learning, its social prestige, all are factors facilitating this. When the profession refuses recognition to some aspiring new healing cult, this brings back memories of childish experiences, when the father frowned upon youthful demands and pretensions.

---

[1] " He was very argumentative, and always wanted proof of anything rather than an accepted opinion. Anything that could be demonstrated he was ready to accept ; but he would combat what could not be proved with all his energy rather than admit it as a truth." Quimby (G. A.), in *New England Magazine*, March, 1888, quoted by Dresser (Anneita G.), *Philosophy of P. P. Quimby* (Boston, 1895), p. 12.

[2] " When quite a child, we . . . passed most of our early years in hunger, pain, weakness and starvation. . . . After years of suffering . . . we made up our mind to die, our doctors kindly assuring us this was our only alternative." Eddy (Mrs M. A. M. B. P. G.), *Science and Health* (Jerusalem, 1924), p. 190.

[3] " M. Coué . . . was delicate during his infancy and boyhood." Noble (Lady), *M. Coué and Auto-Suggestion* (Chatham, London, 1924), p. 1.

Expressions of such an attitude of personal animosity are not far to seek in the writings of P. P. Quimby :

> " I never try to convince a patient that his trouble arises from calomel or any other poison, but the poison of the doctor's opinion in admitting a disease."[1]

Of one of his female patients, he makes the diagnosis :

> " A physician . . . in his ignorance, gave her these words full of poison : ' Your trouble is a cancer in the breast . . . '
> " ' I will admit the swelling,' said I, ' but it is of your own make. You received the seed from the doctor, and he prepared the mind, or matter, for its growth ; but the fruit is the work of the medical faculty '."[2]

The expression, *received the seed from the doctor*, is almost sufficient in itself to establish that the physician is regarded as successor to the once rivaling father, who forced his seed on the mother.

Now we will consider another interesting paragraph :

> " The people, like the children of Israel . . . have lost their way and fallen among strangers or doctors . . . Like Moses, I enter this land and lead them out, and as I pass through the sea of blood or beliefs of these blind guides, I feed them with the bread of wisdom and smite the rock of truth and the water of wisdom gushes out."[3]

Here, it will be seen, Quimby aspires himself to usurp, as a Moses, the father's place, in the same act by which the wicked doctors are dismissed.

He has, moreover, only contempt for sons who adhere to their father instead of joining the standard of revolt :

> " Of all mean-looking things, a human being that is completely under the medical faculty is the lowest. He is

---

[1] Quimby (P. P.), in letter published in *Advertiser*, Portland, Me., February 13th, 1862.

[2] *Quimby MSS.*, 1864. See Dresser (A. G.), *Philosophy of P. P. Quimby*, p. 97.

[3] Quimby (P. P.), see Dresser (H. W.), *Quimby MSS.*, pp. 333-4.

as much a slave as the negro at the South, and, in fact, more so."[1]

Quimby bequeathed, as we shall now see, this antagonism to doctor-fathers, to Trine and other successors.

Statements by R. W. Trine and by some sceptics

A wish to make out a good case for the control of matter by mind, and so to get the better of the doctor-fathers, aided perhaps by an antagonism to the criminal as also a father-surrogate, may be responsible for the following statement by Ralph Waldo Trine. It will come as news to both criminologists and physiological psychologists how easily guilt can be detected:

> " Says a noted American . . . graduate of one of our greatest medical schools . . . ' It has been discovered by scientists that there is a chemical difference between that sudden cold exudation of a person under a deep sense of guilt and the ordinary perspiration ; and the state of the mind can sometimes be determined by chemical analysis of the perspiration of a criminal, which, when brought into contact with selenic acid, produces a distinctive pink colour '."[2]

So far, we have dealt only with the way in which the Œdipus Complex may be presumed to have acted to destroy the confidence of Quimby and those who further developed his ideas, in certain particular old beliefs. But in some persons this complex actually aids in the creation of gods, even while in others the anti-father motive sweeps away the fabric of theology bodily.

C. Moxon found that:

> " The impulses to the creation of a father God are not only the conscious feelings of inferiority, incapacity, and the fear caused by hard times and lack of earthly love, but chiefly the unconscious feeling that one's actual father is

---

[1] *Quimby MSS.*, November, 1861. Dresser (A. G.), *Philosophy of P. P. Quimby*, p. 100.
[2] Trine (R. W.), *In Tune With the Infinite* (London, 1923), pp. 33-4.

all too human, the desire for an ideal lover on whom one may project one's will to power, and the need of a refuge in the transcendental family of God."[1]

In the cases of most extreme detestation of the father, the son is apt to reject theological beliefs altogether. What vitriolic criticism of his father Thomas Hardy has put into some of his poetry ! Take these stanzas from *Nature's Awakening :*

> " Has some Vast Imbecility,
> Mighty to build and blend,
> But impotent to tend,
> Framed us in jest, and left us now in hazardy ?

> " Or come we of an Automaton
> Unconscious of our pains ? . . .
> Or are we live remains
> Of Godhead dying downwards, brain and eye now gone ? "

" Or consider ", as a writer in *The Freethinker* suggests, " the poem in which he asks God ' Why shaped you us ? ' then puts into the mouth of Deity the following reply :

> " . . . My labours—logicless—
> You may explain ; not I.
> Sense-sealed I have wrought, without a guess
> That I evolved a Consciousness
> To ask for reasons why.

> " Strange that ephemeral creatures, who
> By my own ordering are,
> Should see the shortness of my view,
> Use ethic tests I never knew,
> Or made provision for ! "[2]

It is in intellectual and logical qualities that the father is presumed to excel ; whence the peculiar point in calling him imbecile and logicless.

---

[1] Moxon (C.), "A Psycho-Analytic Interpretation of the Christian Creed " *The International Journal of Psycho-Analysis*, vol. II, 1921, p. 56.
[2] Thompson (W.), in *The Freethinker*, London, August 23rd, 1925.

Here I will bring this second chapter of our thesis to an end. I have endeavoured in it to show that the resentment against the father as an oppressor, etc., has played probably a certain part in determining the views of Kenyon, Marx, Hyndman, Humbolt, Paine, Shelley, Emerson, Bentham, Philpotts, Quimby, Mrs Eddy, Hardy, the subject Oriental peoples and our own pacifists.

CHAPTER III

THE FATHER AS MONOPOLIST-CAPITALIST

INTRODUCTORY REMARKS

IN the experience of small children, opulence is represented by the parents, who have ultimate ownership of all the property in their small world. Poverty and dependence are represented by the children, who hold the little they do have, subject to the pleasure of their elders. The father, especially, in their eyes, is a person of unlimited means. They have so little, and he, by comparison, so much. He becomes, therefore, the archetype of the capitalist.

The father is generally the one who first inculcates the virtue of *thrift*. It is, therefore, natural to find that bankers, the personification of the thrift ideal in the community, play decidedly a father rôle. Along with thrift, *industry*, too, is a trait associated with, and praised by, the fathers.

If the latter themselves have practised these virtues, then the oncoming of venerable years generally finds them arrived at the social prestige which goes with the possession of wealth. Thus private property, both as a possession and as a social institution, is an effective means of demarcating the older generation (who have achieved) from the (still only aspiring) younger one.

To the child everything seems to have been arranged for the parents ; and most especially does the boy find a contrast between the way in which his father is able to command the property and even the persons of all the members of the family, and the short shrift with which his own wishes are often met.　All this arouses in him a sense of great injustice.

With the topic of justice a sore spot in his make-up, he grows up in a world full of occurrences which stir his sympathy for the oppressed (children) and rouse his ire against their oppressors (fathers).

The capitalist appears to such an one as a copy of the father.　The landlord in Latin countries is actually called a *patron*.　Bankers, manufacturers (creators) and the whole possessing class are inevitably thought of in terms of the father.　The institution of property is a father-device, which the children clamour to have modified.　Since the propertied class nearly always also is the ruling class, the attitude towards it is over-determined.

Throughout this chapter, therefore, we shall find the old hostility against the father bursting forth as revolt against upper-class manners and virtues and against obedience to paternal figures.

ECONOMICO-POLITICAL TYPE

Value, said Marx, is not a question of supply and demand, but of how much labour went into the product.

Now we look in vain to find such a theory of value actually acted upon, *outside the nursery*.　If you are a truck farmer, you may put in no end of labour in harvesting your vegetables ; but if the market is so glutted that vegetables are rotting on the stalls for lack of buyers, their value is not a whit greater for all your pains.　But in the nursery, the child is rewarded if he has been good and performed his task dutifully, although no one wants his product.

It is therefore by a reversion to childhood, that a communist magazine makes the identification :

" Value and labour are two words that have the same meaning."[1]

From such a position it is only a further step to declare that the saving of one's product at all is a silly procedure, which we unwillingly do only to please our parents—a statement having not the remotest relation to the realities of adult life, but entirely true in babyhood. This topic comes most properly under the head of anal erotism, which is foreign to my thesis. But we may consider here a formulation by John Burns, which obviously involves hostility to exploiting fathers (capitalist rogues) :

" Thrift was invented by capitalistic rogues to beguile fools to destruction, and to deprive honest fools of their diet and their proper comfort."[2]

At least one socialist writer extends this ban to cover both temperance and industry as well. His fantastic statement may well represent a revolt, not only against the inhibitions of certain pleasures of infancy, but against also the insistences of that important father-surrogate, the schoolmaster. These are his words :

" Temperance, thrift, industry, only serve to make labour an easier or more valuable prey to capital. If they reduce the cost of living in any particular they but reduce the cost of labour to the capitalist."[3]

Perhaps it is only fair to this writer to say that he doubtless would confine the implications of his remark to the present social order, and assume that a new set of

---

[1] *The Plebs.* (Oxford, November, 1918), vol. X, no. 10, p. 228.

[2] Burns (John, M.P.), to the Trade Union Congress, at Norwich : *Report of the 27th Annual Trade Union Congress,* p. 55. Cited in *Anti-Socialist Speakers' Handbook,* p. 253.

[3] Quelch (H.), *Economics of Socialism,* p. 16. Quoted in *Anti-Socialist Speakers' Handbook,* p. 253.

economic laws will apply in a society in which no individual, but the municipality, or the state, is to be the employer.[1]

We should then have the father-loving (pro-state) complex working on the side of the social innovator—unless perhaps the new state is identified with the young hero who is to slay the capitalists and so liberate our mother country.

The topics of crime and immorality figure (as we intimated in Chapter I) very prominently in the arguments of both socialists and anti-socialists. The former say that nearly all crime is caused by the temptations of great wealth, the injustice of its present distribution, and the warping of souls by poverty. The *antis* reply that, on the contrary, it is due to relaxation of discipline which is connected with maudlin sympathy with those who don't deserve it, and to the preaching that laws are made by the ruling class in their own interests.

The socialists say the children are tempted to their downfall by desire to imitate the heartless vanity of their parents, and naturally want their share of the good things of which father and mother seem, according to the newspapers, to have so much. The parents reply that the children would never notice such things, but that their minds are perverted by the pernicious revolutionary ideas.

The sons may preach altruism as a protest against the father's real or alleged egoism, but it is an altruism, which more or less excludes the father himself—it is to benefit those who have been brought together by common interest against him. So far, from *his* view point, it seems a kind of egoism.

Indeed, sons themselves sometimes prefer the term,

---

[1] But one is reminded of Godfrey Elton's rhyme on the soldiers' cemeteries in France :

> " Tell the Professors, you that pass us by,
> They taught Political Economy,
> And here, obedient to its laws, we lie."

egoism. The fathers (teachers, priests, etc.) have always been preaching "altruism" and meaning by the word, service to themselves—further denial of the interests of youth in obedience to the wise saws of crabbed age. "Enough of this," says youth, "we will have no more altruism ; egoism shall be our watchword. Hereafter we youth will look after ourselves first."

Sinn fein, the name of the rebel Irish movement, as is well known, means "ourselves".

Nietzsche and Stirner are the best known modern proponents of the egoist philosophy, unless we go back to Bentham and the Hedonists. Of their followers who are known to me personally several lead lives of idealistic devotion. But with an interesting obstinacy they insist that no action of their lives is to be attributed to any motive beyond enlightened self-interest.

We may well suppose that a protectionist writer is in rebellion against altruistic preachments of the free-traders, who are thus father-like, and that is why he maintains that by

"each nation . . . regarding its own interests . . . the general interest of the whole human race will be effectually furthered and secured."[1]

Religio Therapeutic Type

A striking fact about Christianity is that in the beginning it was communistic, whereas now the movements called Christianity and Communism are the antitheses of each other.

Early Christianity Communistic

It is coming to be generally recognised that the early Christians were a communist sect. Jesus, rebel against

[1] Byles (J. B.), *Sophisms of Free Trade . . . Examined* (London and New York, 1904), p. 69.

the father-types represented in Scribes, Pharisees, High Priests, etc., was also a rebel against the institution of private property.

He cannot be classed as a socialist in the sense of having a clear-cut plan whereby the masses were to carry on the large processes of industry, secure the services of the capable, and protect themselves alike against their indigent and their exploiting members. Witness his utterances about lilies of the field, birds of the air, and giving no heed to the morrow. But his sect was open to the rich man only on condition of his selling whatever he had and giving to the poor. That this condition was general, and not intended merely to fit the spiritual needs of the one rich young man to whom it was addressed, it is clear from the warning that for the rich to enter heaven was as hard as for a cable ("camel" the older translations make it) to enter the eye of a needle— an impossible accomplishment.[1]

That the early Christians differed from the modern (certain small sects excepted) to the extent of sharing Jesus's attitude, is evidenced by the case of the elders *versus* Ananias and wife.

After the first youthful century or two of democratic and communistic enthusiasm, we find Christianity reconciled to the father figures represented in priests, bishops, and finally a supreme pontifex or "papa". With its recognition by Constantine as the official religion of the Roman State (father par excellence), its tale of martyrs dwindles, and it turns to martyrizing others, burning libraries and heretics. At the same time it relegates the communistic principle to be practised by isolated groups of ascetics. The most communistic of its founders of orders, St Francis, was compelled by a certain ambivalence to remain within the Church's fold, and policy on the latter's part dictated the retention of a saint with so large a following. But the antagonism

---

[1] This whole subject is fully elaborated by Brown (Bishop Mont gommery), *Christianism and Communism*.

between the two was fundamental. Even before St Francis' death, his order was forced by the Pope into betrayal of this troublesome son's essential rule, which was that the order should possess no convents or other property of its own.

Socialist Hostility to Christianity

To-day there are very few Christian sects which regard community of property as being virtuous. Common ownership by all is professed by rebel movements which mostly are not friendly to orthodox religion.

We sometimes find cases where assent to belief in God is denied on grounds which seem economic rather than metaphysical, and therefore logically irrelevant to the point at issue, but in which we can perceive clearly the affect which centres around paternal surrogates like *master* and *boss*. For instance, in a recent debate in New York, one man expostulated in the following terms against religious faith :

" ' Thy will be done ' ; a magnificent democratic motto ! The pious slave who prays ' Thy will be done ' to a master in the skies, will pray ' Thy will be done ' to a master on the earth ! And he who prostrates his manhood before a heavenly boss on Sunday, will prostrate his manhood before an earthly boss on the other days of the week."[1]

Perhaps a more transparent case of the anti-paternal and, derivatively from that, the atheistic, turn which may be given by dislike of the father as monopolist of

[1] Ward (P.), in debate with Nearing (S.). Ward also made the following quotation and comment : " Jesus answered him : ' The first of all commandments is . . . Thou shalt love the Lord thy God with all thy heart, and with all thy soul, and with all thy mind, and with all thy strength ; this is the first commandment. And the second is like, namely this ', (and this is where my friend quotes) : ' Thou shalt love thy neighbour as thyself '. Eight lines to God and two to your neighbour. I wish to ask my good friend this : If a man loves God with all his heart, with all his soul, with all his mind, and with all his strength, how much love has he got left for his neighbour ? " In other words, Ward cannot conceive but there must be diversity of interest between father and sons.

F

the family funds, exists in the case of the late H. M. Hyndman. He says :

> " My father . . . laid up for himself treasure in heaven by benefactions of which I, his eldest son, can scarcely in honesty say I approve.[1]

> " My father himself early developed a turn for expenditure and charity, which, I regret to say, was not accompanied by a . . . talent for acquisition. He had neither the initiative and ability of his own father, nor the revolutionary turn of the man of '98, being, in fact, I believe, a member of the Conservative Club, and a supporter of the Tory Party."[2]

A fact to which infidels never tire in calling attention is that the churches are regularly on the side of property, entrenched privilege and the oppressor :

> " The unproductive labourers are now employed in giving a false direction to the egoism of the subjected classes, and in perverting the calculation upon which it is based.   This is effected by setting up a fanciful moral sanction over and against the labourer's revolutionary tendencies, causing the disinherited classes to dread the idea of revolt, and to look upon rebellion as more abhorrent even than submission. In this way the bearing of the proletarians towards their masters . . . comes under the discipline of a moral law, which is exactly calculated to prevent their egoism and render them tolerant under capitalist usurpation."[3]

Followers of some of the younger and more liberal cults may deny that this needs to be so.   Yet there is a good psychological reason why we should expect it, if as is here maintained, all these conservative institutions alike tend chiefly to enlist the father-minded type of individual.

The whole conservative policy is abhorrent to the sons who have declared war against the fathers, and who,

---

[1] Hyndman (H. M.), *Record of an Adventurous Life* (London, 1911), pp. 1-2.
[2] *Ibid*, pp. 6-7.
[3] Loria (Achille), *Economic Foundations of Society*, p. 20, quoted by E. & C. P. in *The Plebs*, Oxford, vol. X, p. 135.

when the latter ask for a truce, delight in denying it to them in their own phrases, thus :

" A line for industrial pacifists :
  " Woe to him who seeks to pour oil upon the waters when God hath brewed them into a gale '."[1]

In this chapter of our thesis (to sum up) we have seen how jealousy of the father as monopolist and capitalist, led to quarrels with him over standards of morals, altruism, etc., and to antagonism against religion and eligious bequests in several cases.

[1] " Moby Dick "—Cover of *The Plebs*, Oxford, 1922, vol. XIV, no. 9.

CHAPTER IV

THE CASTRATING OR KILLING PHANTASY

INTRODUCTORY REMARKS

ONE of the discoveries made by Freud in probing the minds of his patients (a discovery that has met with fierce opposition) is what he calls the castration complex. Little boys frequently are threatened by nursemaids or others with amputation of their male organ unless they stop playing with it. Colour is given to the possibility of such punishment being carried out, by occasional sight of the genitals of girls, which appear to the boy to have been bereft of their interesting member.

The experiences of Dr Melanie Klein in analysing young children[1] convinced her that young children who never had a chance of observing coitus have nevertheless a vague intuitive apprehension of what takes place between their parents. In any case, the evidence goes to show that nature has equipped the child with an intensity of interest in genital matters which immensely quickens its perception, and also with other elements, as yet undefined, of a " set " in the direction of interpreting such perceptions correctly to a degree which is uncanny.

Whatever may prove to be the ultimate explanation, the small boy correctly associates (such is the finding of Frau Klein and other analysts) the genital organs with the antagonism between himself and his father. He feels that, for his evil wishes towards the father, an

[1] Related by her to members of the British Psycho-Analytic Society in July, 1925.

appropriate punishment would be for the father to do what nurse sometimes threatened to, namely emasculate him.

An example of the castration complex is given by Pfister in the case of a boy who " expressed a wish to cut off his father's nose ". The associations given by the boy showed that *nose* was a substitute for *penis*.[1]

While, as in this instance, the desire is to perform the operation on someone else (and the person is probably always either the father or a father-substitute) it may be regarded as the expression of sexual jealousy.

We shall now find it worth while to discuss the imposition of secrecy as a special symbol of castration, and, afterwards, the special rôle of this in the professions to-day.

Imposed Silence or Secrecy as Castration

It seems that one of the particular forms assumed by the castration-complex is that of compulsory silence. The researches of Dr Bryan, Dr Jones and Mr Flügel may be referred to in this connection.

Dr Douglas Bryan has described the case of a patient in whom loss of speech represented an unwitting phantasy that his father was punishing him by cutting off his penis —when the patient discovered this meaning to himself, the loss of speech disappeared.[2]

Secrecy, when part of the tactics employed by the parents in sexual matters especially, to keep the younger generation in their place, is disliked by the juniors. In

---

[1] Pfister (O.), *Love in Children*, transl. Paul (London, 1924), p. 286.

[2] " In the patient's own written words : ' My father has cut off my penis with my mother's vulva for usurping his privilege of entering it, and has therefore deprived me of my voice—which is absurd, therefore my voice should return, and does ! At this moment he speaks '
" During the analysis next day, the patient suddenly remarked : ' I am not really speaking with my voice, but with my mind only '. Here was an obvious self-castration, which he quickly recognized." Bryan (Dr D.), " Speech and Castration ", in *Int. Jour. of Psycho-Analysis*, July, 1925, vol. VI, part 3, pp. 317-23.

their own turn these generally elect to practice the same tactics upon their parents.

" Secrecy . . . and spying . . . are certainly derived from forbidden curiosity about secret, i.e. sexual, matters in early childhood."[1]

Dr Ernest Jones, in his essay on the " Madonna's Conception Through the Ear ",[2] shows how speech is the equivalent of life, creative power and God (Logos doctrine). The tongue represents the phallus. Gaseous fertilization, especially, is the antithesis of castration. J. C. Flügel, in an article on the International Language movement, further develops these ideas.[3]

[1] Jones (E.), " A Psycho-Analytic Study of Hamlet," in his *Essays in Applied Psycho-Analysis*, pp. 269 ff., p. 90.

[2] Jones (E.), *Essays in Applied Psycho-Analysis*, pp. 269 ff.

[3] He mentions the cutting off of tongues of criminals in Byzantium and England as having been carried out *pari passu* with such known castration displacements as blinding and cutting off the hands, as well as with actual castration itself. Tongues of animals were used as amulets for good luck, strength, knowledge, and eloquence—all but the last being equivalents of sexual potency.

In Bohemia, he continues, the tongue of a male snake, torn from the living animal (castration) on St George's Eve (St George being the dragon-slayer or father-castrator), when placed under the tongue will give eloquence. The Arjunta pierce the tongue to initiate medicine men, who must be magically eloquent. Tongues were sacrificed to Hermes, god of eloquence, money, commerce, music and winds.

Not only speech, but the very understanding of language is shown by Flügel to have a phallic significance, since there is a belief that the language of animals is learnt by eating serpents. The animal in his totemic significance means the father. Some Shamans in North America are initiated by means of a dream in which an animal teaches them the animal language. There are many stories in which the language of animals helps a boy to rise to power, humiliate his father and marry the princess. The young child would associate language with other superior powers of adults. Stammering is associated with inferiority (and castration ?). The " impotence " of a laryngitis patient of Flügel's own proved to be a castration-complex.

Naturally, if speech and understanding are symbols of potency, we may expect to find that silence and secrecy are castration symbols. Jones, in the Madonna Essay alluded to above, shows how dumbness is the equivalent of impotence and death.

That silence is the symbolic equivalent of chastity is shown, argues Flügel, by the customs of the seclusion of women about the time of puberty (the analogue of the initiations of men) or during early widowhood, or as a bride and toward other men during the early years of marriage. In Sardinia, lovers talk only with their hands. In Thuringia, yellow mullen is dug in silence on Midsummer eve (the eve of magic potency derived from the sexual). In some tribes of Western

Secrecy is the characteristic attribute of those who pretend to occult knowledge, i.e. to being initiated into wisdom too exalted for less mature mortals.[1] From earliest times, the rule of silence has been imposed by groups of initiates :

" Unless one is an initiated member of Australian society, it is impossible to learn the jealously-guarded tribal secrets. The native is as secretive as a freemason."[2]

In Buddhist Tantrism, " secret rites are the business of a few ' devotees '."[3]

The same rule of silence (symbolic castration) was in vogue with the ancient Pythagorean Brotherhood. Their saying, " Speak not about Pythagorean concerns without light ",[4] imposed a long initiation of silence upon the younger members, besides serving to enshroud the order in the glamour of parent-like secrecy.[5]

Care was taken, moreover, to admit only desirable

Victoria it is forbidden to marry a wife who speaks the same dialect as oneself. In some places there are differences between the language as spoken by men and by women.

Flügel further recalls how Lorenz, in his study of the Titan Motive, shows that the Babel story belongs to the class of legends concerned with the storming of Heaven. According to Hygenus, further, Hermes, the God of winds, is responsible for discord and diversity of speech among men. In Polynesian versions of the Titan story, the wind god, Tawhirima-tea, assists his parents and scatters his brothers. All these are variations of the theme of dismemberment. The Pentecostal gift of tongues (glossolalia, not zeno glossia) is the providential antithesis to Babel. Glossalia as a religious phenomenon, has been studied by Pfister. Here God as the Holy Ghost is endowing man with some of his own creative power. See Flügel (J. C.), *Internat. Jl. of Psycho-Analysis*, London, 1924, vol. I.

[1] Jones (E.), " A Psycho-Analytic Study of Hamlet " in *Essays in Applied-Psychology*, p. 208.

[2] James (E. O.), *Primitive Ritual and Belief*, p. 27.

[3] Poussin (de la Valleé), article " Tantrism " in *Encylo. of Religion and Ethics*.

[4] Iamblicus, *Pythagorean Symbols with Explanations*, pp. 80-1.

[5] " Early in the course came a long period of silence, in which the neophyte conformed his life to the rules of physical and moral training laid down for him, without presuming to teach others except by example. It is probable that a large proportion of the members advanced no further than this stage.

" Pythagoras left no writings. Our knowledge of his teachings and institutions depends on the traditions of his disciples." Harrison (F.), *New Calendar*, p. 107.

applicants, and such as would be likely to remain loyal, according to the admonition, " Receive not a swallow into your house ".[1]

" The followers of Pythagoras . . . imposed, out of respect for their divine character, a ritual of silence on themselves. For many were the divine and ineffable secrets which they had heard, but which it was difficult for any to keep who had not previously learnt that silence also is a mode of speech."[2]

Pythagoras also advises us to "obliterate the mark of the pot from the ashes ", and this is explained by Iamblicus as meaning we should :

" . . . consign to oblivion the confusion and grossness which subsist in corporeal and sensible demonstrations . . . But ashes are here assumed instead of the dust in the tables, in which the Pythagoreans completed their demonstrations."[3]

The notion of breaking cleanly with one's past origin is thus implied in the Pythagorean maxim. But to break with our origin is suspiciously like breaking with our ancestry. At the same time, that Pythagorean admonition implies a wish to be *secretive* about our origin.

One means, long ago discovered, of preserving the secrecy of any cult or craft, is the employment of a technical jargon, as the Sufis, according to Claude Field,

" make use of certain technical expressions. Of these Ghazzali has treated in Ibya-ul-Ulum."[4]

---

[1] Iamblicus (*Pythagorean Symbols with Explanations*, p. 98) interprets this as meaning : " Do not admit to your homes a man who is indolent. . . . It uses the swallow as an image of indolence, and an interruption of time, because this bird visits us for a certain part of the year, and for a short time becomes as it were our guest ; but it leaves us for the greater part of the year ". In any case, admission was difficult and provisional, and long initiation was a pre-requisite.

[2] Philostratus, *Life of Appolonius of Tyana*, transl. F. C. Conybeare, vol. I, p. 5.

[3] *Pythagorean Symbols with Explanations by Iamblicus*, p. 113.

[4] Field (Claude), *Mystics and Saints of Islam*. Appendix II. *A Mohammedan Exposition of Sufism*, by Ibu Khaldoun, p. 198.

and Nicholson mentions that these Sufis

> "regarded themselves as a peculiarly favoured class, possessing an esoretic knowledge of the Qu'ran, and the Apostolic traditions, and using technical expressions which no ordinary Muslim could understand."[1]

We are not surprised then that

> "Admission to the order was obtained through a long and systematic course of training ; and it would seem that there were at least two stages of membership before complete initiation was reached."[2]

The same cautiousness in admitting new candidates, and the same severity of apprenticeship, was in vogue among the Essenes, a sect whom some regard as the source of the ethics of Jesus, and so of Christianity so far as that is derived from him :

> "Excluded from the Temple in Jerusalem, the Essenes formed a community resembling that of a monastic order, entrance into which involved a double novitiate. An applicant spent a year outside the Community, during which its mode of life was recommended to him. He was provided with a spade (symbol of work), an apron (to be used at the ablutions), and a white dress (the robe of the order). During his second novitiate of two years the candidate was admitted to the lustrations but not to the meals. At the end of that period he was admitted to the order. But before becoming a full member, he had to bind himself by a solemn oath (the last permitted to him, since the Essenes rejected the use of the oath elsewhere) in which he promised to honour God, to exercise justice, to injure no one intentionally, to obey the superiors, and not to divulge any of the secrets of the order."[3]

This group appears to have been peculiarly suspicious of youth :

> "There is among the Essenes no mere child, not even a scarce bearded lad, or young man, since of such as these

---

[1] Nicholson (R. A.), in article " Sufis " in *Encyclopædia of Religion and Ethics.*
[2] Harrison (F.), *New Calendar*, p. 107.
[3] Uhlhorn (G.), in article " Essenes " in new Schaff-Herzog *Encyclopædia of Religious Knowledge.*

the moral dispositions are unstable and apt to change in accordance with their imperfect age ; they are all full grown men, already verging upon old age, as being no longer swept away by the flood of bodily impulses, or led by their passions, but in the enjoyment of the genuine and only liberty."[1]

Many religious bodies have carried down to the present day this tradition of secrecy and difficult initiation. Among them, the Sufis deserve particularly to be mentioned, because of the vow of obedience required to the father-figure.

" It was generally held that for those entering on the religious life a teacher was indispensable . . . The authority of the *Shaikhs* was absolute. It lay with them to decide whether the novice, after his probationary period, should be granted leave to take the vow of obedience to his master which was exacted from all candidates for initiation. Hujiwiri mentions a three years probation.[2]

" The neophyte (murid, " willer ", " intender ") has been put through a longer or shorter process of initiation, in some forms of which it is plain that he is brought under hypnotic control by his instructor and put into rapport with him."[3]

Further to emphasize the esoteric nature of his teachings, a cult founder named Gurdiev Georgiadis uses the same cultish device as with the Sufis is followed, of employing a special vocabulary of technical terms, e.g. by the word " hydrogen ", reference is understood to the suppositious series of similar existences, organs or substances, throughout the alleged plural universes, to which are assigned certain numbers or rates of " vibra-

---

[1] Philo, *Apology for the Jews*, excerpted in *Enc. Praep Ey*, vol. VIII, 11 (ed. E. H. Gifford, 1903) quoted by J. Moffatt in article " Essenes " in *Encyclopædia of Religion and Ethics*.
[2] Nicholson (R. A.), article of " Sufis " in *Encyclopædia of Religion and Ethics*.
[3] MacDonald (D. B.), article " Derwish " in *Encyclopædia of Islam*.

tion ", calculated in a peculiar way, and multiples of each other.[1]

At the Institute Gurdiev for the Harmonic Development of Man, a scientific occidental mind is unfavourably impressed by an unwillingness to answer questions unless they are couched in terms which seem to the master to indicate that the questioner has progressed a certain way along the mystical path. I understand that this is all in strict accord with certain esoteric traditions. One can, also, appreciate some strength in the arguments advanced in its favour. It is none the less difficult to dismiss a feeling of quackishness about this assumption of paternal inscrutability and of possessing great secrets which will be revealed only when the little son has matured.[2]

[1] No attempt is made to propagate these beliefs, apart from the general recruiting for the institute. This last is done by members interesting their friends in it, and also by Mr Gurdiev's representatives such as Ouspensky in England, and Orage in America.
This fact is consistent with both the " esoteric tradition ", and the special emphasis which Gurdiev places upon discipline as against intellection.

[2] Behind such an attitude, one of course suspects an uncertainty on the part of the teacher of being able to defend his theory in the open field against a competent adversary. But the contrary position was defended by a doctor at the institute, to whom I had confided my views.
" I used ", he told me, " to be a lecturer on certain phases of medicine, at the University of Petrograd. At the end of my course, there were always a certain number of students who asked the privilege of working in my laboratory. I found it better, instead of encouraging many of them, to raise the greatest number of possible objections and obstacles. Thus only the most earnest ones would come."
I answered that, admitting that the principle might hold in special cases, yet the man who assumed the rôle of a cult leader seemed rather to have taken on responsibilities similar to those of, say, a superintendent of public instruction. If such a man deemed that the children of the community ought to have more adequate knowledge of hygiene, he would hardly accomplish his purpose by making it hard for any except the most persistent, and those only after months or years of application, to get any facts. A more effective way would be to open numerous hygiene classes and to stimulate the amount of attendance and explicitness of instruction.
To this my doctor friend could only reply that Gurdiev's present task was that of training his assistants. Only after this was completed could the question of public instruction come up.

If we are to avoid calling them deliberate charlatans, therefore—and this would be in some cases unjust— we must suppose that the founders of the occult and esoteric societies have a strongly developed complex impelling secrecy. This may in some cases be connected with childish scoptophilia and reaction against the deceptions of parents—a subject not to be treated of here. In other cases we shall suspect it is a phase of sympathy felt toward the parent himself. This will appear the more probable when the general attitude is a religious[1] or otherwise authoritarian one. But I invite consideration of the suggestion that while the rule

Yet this " arcane " knowledge, possession of which is accredited to men of the type of Gurdiev, is assumed to have been handed down through these esoteric schools from fathers living milleniums ago. One inclines to ask how much longer the public must wait for the training of these assistants.

[1] Gurdievism is not wholly (in, at any rate, the usual sense) a religion. If we call it a cult, we must append the adjective metaphysical rather than religious, and we must allow also that the system of metaphysics it espouses is held to be of very indifferent importance : " Live the life and ye shall know the doctrine." It is held that when the mind is reformed by the cult exercises, it becomes capable of perceiving instinctively the truth of an extraordinary system of cosmology.

This system is hardly worthy of serious consideration, since its only " proof " is the assumption of correspondences of objective reality to the structure of the mind as it is alleged to be perceived by those who have attained a necessary degree of self development. Moreover, Mr Ouspensky, who has become a disciple of Gurdiev, and who previously wrote a book, _Tertium Organum_, setting forth a similar system, is now about to publish another more orthodox and up-to-date presentation of the subject. In bare outlines, this cosmology is as follows :

Over our known world of three-dimensional space is set another of four dimensions ; over that, one of five ; over that, one of six ; and over that, one of seven dimensions, which is " the absolute ". The beings which exist in the universe of more dimensions are " higher " than those existing in the lower, and control to a great extent their destinies. They also live at a slower rate, which we can calculate according to this law ; that the life time of an earthly creature is the time of a single breath for an analogous creature in the next higher existence, and is the time taken for the mere winking of an eye by an analogous creature on a plane higher still, etc.

I suggest that we have thus in these suppositious creatures a series of father-_imagos_ growing more and more imposing as they recede into the background. They correspond to the ancestral traditions of primitive people, in which the progenitors of a clan are regarded with increasing awe according to their earlier dates, until the first of them all are given the rank of gods. May we not suppose that the more remote in such a series, represent the child's more remote memories of his father ; who appeared most omnipotent when the child was youngest ?

of silence gratifies these motivations, it also serves as a symbolic castration, punishing on the one hand oneself[1] but on the other hand particularly the novices and new initiates. And I call attention to the hatred shown generally by outsiders toward a secret society in their community. Does not this seem to imply a general intuitive appreciation of the castratory wishes symbolized by secrecy ? The sons resent their exclusion and symbolic castration.

In the Professions To-day

By their penchant for secrecy, many contemporary social groups reveal how they sense themselves as fathers.

The most outstanding examples are, of course, mystical or sacredotal fraternities. Priests even take on the titles of Father, *Papa* (Pope), etc. The next worst offenders are the medical men, the older school of whom were especially strong on keeping patients ignorant of the method of their treatment. Prescriptions are still written in code. But all learned professions affect technical terms and an erudite lingo. Behind this attitude, an onlooker seems to sense the desire of the group for the position of fathers in the community. Other conduct of the group is generally present to confirm such an inference.

Probational periods and associate-memberships are in effect modified forms of initiation ; esoteric doctrines also serve to keep out the sons. In most learned societies, candidates are expected to have at least mastered the technical jargon of the group. The British Psycho-Analytic Society requires every applicant first of all to have been analysed. After this often very painful preliminary ordeal lasting from six months to two years, he may be proposed as an associate member of the society. The associate now absorbs more of the wisdom of the elders and may also advance himself by

[1] We shall treat of self-punishment in Part Two, chapter I,

performance of merit-bringing labours, such as contributing reviews and papers, until at length he is admitted to full membership on a par with the fathers. In some foreign countries, as Germany and the United States, an additional pre-requisite is the having a medical degree (we elsewhere discuss the peculiarly paternal meaning conferred by this degree).

Against these tendencies on the part of learned societies one may always find groups of sons leagued in rebellion—protestant cults, societies for medical freedom, and what not.

ECONOMICO-POLITICAL TYPE

The older generation, class-conscious of themselves as elders or fathers, intuitively perceive in co-operative, democratic and socialistic movements, a revolt of youth against their authority. So they seek to cut off the power of the young through censorship, whilst the young find another symbol for reciprocal fantasies in programmes of catastrophic reform, as we shall presently see.

Censorship

The perception by the elders that these movements are a revolt against their domination leads them to measures of suppression which often are unwisely passionate and instinctive. They censor the public's reading and thinking as a father prescribes for his child. Their intolerance quite " gives them away "—and fires opposition.

> " A survey of the restrictions on teaching in schools and colleges just completed by the American Civil Liberties Union, shows that more restrictive laws have been passed during the last six months than at any time in American history. These laws prohibit the teaching of evolution,

require compulsory reading of the Bible, and forbid the
employment of radical or pacifist teachers."[1]

[1] " The survey shows that Congress passed one such law as a rider
to the 1925 appropriation bill for the district of Columbia, providing
' that no part of this sum shall be available for the payment of the
salary ' of any educational director ' who permits the teaching of
partizan politics, disrespect of the Holy Bible, or that ours is an inferior
form of government '. This law is now in force in the District of
Columbia.

  " Pensylvania, Ohio, Delaware, West Virginia, and Kentucky, have
laws requiring the daily reading of the Bible in public schools ' without
comment ', and providing for the discharge and revocation of the
certificate of a teacher who does not conform to the act. Similar
bills have been introduced in the legislatures of Virginia, Texas, New
Jersey, and Washington. A test of this type of statute was made in
South Dakota in March, where Judge McNenny ruled that a school-
board has the authority to expel high school students who leave the
class room during Bible reading. Thirteen students were expelled. . . .

  " The first state law prohibiting the teaching of the doctrine of
evolution in public schools and colleges was passed in Tennessee in
March. Resolutions of State Boards forbidding the teaching of evolution were previously adopted in North Carolina and Florida.

  " Missouri state colleges and schools are forbidden by a rider to
the appropriation bill, recently passed, to employ any person ' who
teaches, or advocates in public or private that the citizens of this State
should not protect the Government of the United States from aggression
by other nations '. In the recent Ohio legislature a resolution was
introduced authorizing an investigation of members of the faculties
of three State universities, with the object of ousting ' radicals and
atheists '." *Press Service of the American Civil Liberties Union*, New
York, April, 28th, 1925, Bulletin, no. 152. The term " professional
patriot " refers to those persons who subsidise military or naval propaganda because they stand to reap a profit from government contracts.
The above quotation must, however, be now somewhat modified.
The same Press service reported, on May 13th, 1925 :—

  " Significant indications of better conditions for civil liberties, as
reported by the American Civil Liberties Union in its survey for the
month of April, are the veto of the compulsory Bible reading bill in
Ohio, the defeat of the state constabulary bill in the same state and
the final blow to the Kansas Industrial Court by the U.S. Supreme
Court. Attacks on radicals celebrating May Day were fewer than at
any time in recent years. Mob violence, however, is reported from
widely separate areas, with seven fresh cases, two by the Klan, and
one by Klan opponents.

  " Two cases of unusual interest are noted in the Union's survey,
the convictions of the two soldiers at Honolulu for their communist
views, with excessive sentences of 40 and 26 years, and the sentencing
of Roger N. Baldwin, director of the Civil Liberties Union to six months
for arranging a free speech meeting during the Paterson silk strike.

  " The situation in California remains unchanged except for an
interesting suit brought by I.W.W. publications against restrictions
under the Busick injunction, the Union states. The attack on two
Harvard magazines for alleged ' indecent matter ' aroused widespread
interest. The Post Office Department refused to bar them from mails.
Old issues of civil rights in West Virginia have cropped out again with
an indication that the organized miners are likely to get more rights
than they have had,"

How easily mere verbal guarantees of free speech, i.e. equal potency of sons with the father, whether written in a constitution or embodied in local tradition, are evaded when not backed by any real appreciation of the need of occasionally challenging the rule of the father, is shown by the casuistical distinctions now current in America between liberty and " license ". This was expressed even some decades ago by Anthony Comstock :

" There is a wide difference between the patriot's liberty and the Liberal's so-called liberty—license."[1]

But we are here concerned with the conduct of the fathers less for its own sake, than as it shall prove provocative to the sons. And actually it is easy to observe how it does fill them with hate and zeal. Against restrictions on speech which have been alluded to above, one of the sons' confederacies, the American Civil Liberties Union, announces that :

" Efforts to get court action on all these restrictive laws will be made through our attorneys. The constitutional guarantees of separation of church and state, it is believed, offers a ground for contesting the laws requiring Bible reading. The U.S. Supreme Court already has before it one restrictive school law passed in Oregon and aimed at abolishing the parochial schools."[2]

When the interference of the governent with private affairs touches upon the matter of freedom of speech, the protest of the rebel sons is particularly vigorous.

---

[1] Comstock (A.), *Traps for the Young* (New York, 1884), p. 237.
[2] The Union then points out the hated father figures who are behind the various measures :
" The chief sources of inspiration for this new and unprecedented crop of gag laws on teaching are the Klu Klux Klan, the Fundamentalists, and the professional patriotic societies. The Klan is back of the compulsory Bible reading and anti-parochial school laws, the Fundamentalists back of the anti-evolution bills, and the professional patriots back of the anti-radical and anti-pacifist measures." *Press Service*, American Civil Liberties Union, New York, April 28th, 1925 ; bulletin no, 52.

We shall the better understand why this is so when we have examined the special complexes involved when speech is cut off, and how these go back to feelings connected with the superior potency of the father. Investigations by Ernest Jones establish a presumption that interest in sounds is in large measure traceable to childish concern with paternal flatus.[1]

In the essay in which he records this (the essay on the Madonna's Conception) he shows how speech=life, creative power and God (Logos doctrine), how tongue= phallus, and gaseous fertilization=antithesis of castration. Whence dumbness=death or impotence.

Censorship, therefore, means symbolic castration by the father. The sons resent this with due heat, and demand Free Speech, the symbol of equal potency with the father.

Therefore, the attitude of the sons towards censorship will, in general, be determined by their castration complexes. Those who have a strong unwitting fear of this talion-measure on the part of their fathers, will be most exercised over the attempt to emasculate their speech. So important did this issue seem to the founders of the United States (late rebels against King and English father-land) that they embodied the principle in their first amendment to the Constitution of the United States :

> " Congress shall pass no law abridging the freedom of speech and press, or of the right of the people peacefully to assemble."

[1] Jones (E.), " The Madonna's Conception ", in his *Essays in Applied Psycho-Analysis*, pp. 284-5. He also shows how intimately speech, through breath, is associated with the same paternal source.
" Speech was therefore quite naturally considered identical with God, i.e. the Creator, and the doctrine of the Logos has played a prominent part in most of the higher religions. . . . The association between the Holy Ghost and speech was just as intimate ; the saints ' spoke by the Holy Ghost ' (St Mark, XII, 36 ; Acts of the Apostles, XIII, 2 ; XVI, 7), or were '.filled by the Holy Ghost and prophesied ' (St Luke, I, 67). . . ." Jones (E.), " The Madonna's Conception ". Publ. in *Jahrbuch der Psycho-Analyse*, 1914, Band. VI. ; republished in his *Essays on Applied Psycho-Analysis* (1923), p. 288.

G

and this amendment has been made the basis of decision by the Supreme Court.[1]

During the. Great War, these guarantees in America, as elsewhere, collapsed before the intensity of official fervour and of mob feeling. Even a rather Conservative paper was moved to protest when *The Nation* was excluded from the mails for an editorial which criticized the mission of Samuel Gompers to England :

> " The people have a right to think even in war . . . It is time now to make an end of the new process of Prussianization . . . under the pretence of super-patriotism." (i.e. super-father-ism.][2]

During this War, organizations like the Civil Liberties Union of New York, with wide-spread branches, came into being. They have since functioned most actively in connection with the many industrial disputes which are the most frequent excuse for the interferences with freedom of speech which characterize America.

In general, the Libertarians insist, with Herbert Spencer, that to resist all interference is, on general principles, a virtue and even an obligation. According to a French liberal :

> " Il faut insister sur vos propres droits, ainsi que sur les droits des autres. La justice est la fondation d'une bonne vie, dont l'edifice superieur est la bonté."[3]

Typical utterances in favour of free speech are such as these :

[1] " To suffer the civil magistrate to intrude his power into the field of opinion, or to restrain the profession or propagation of principles, on supposition of their ill-tendency is a dangerous fallacy, will make his opinions the rule of judgment, and approve or condemn the sentiments of others only as they shall square with, or differ from his own. It is time enough for the rightful purpose of civil government for its officers to interfere when principles break out into overt acts against peace and good order." Virginia Legislature ; approved in *Reynolds vs. United States*, 98, U.S., 163, cited by Vestal in letter published in *The Record*, Los Angeles, May 22nd, 1923.

[2] *The World*, New York, September 22nd, 1918.

[3] Charles (A.), *Les Abeilles Du Bien*.

" Let truth and error grapple. Whoever knew truth
to be beaten in a fair fight ? " (Milton).

" Truth crushed to earth will rise again,
The eternal years of God are hers.
But error, wounded, writhes in pain,
And dies among his worshippers." (Lord Byron).

" If we all agreed finally and for good, talking would be
nonsense. But because we disagree, talking is the part
of wisdom." (Horace Traubal).

" The right to say things necessarily implies the right
to say foolish things. The answer to foolish speech is wise
speech and not force."

" The Republic is founded on the faith that if the American
people are permitted freely to hear foolish and wise speech,
a majority will choose the wise. If that faith is not justified,
the Republic is based upon sand."[1]

In the Miltonian quotation, we get the echo of two
parties " grapple "-ing, and are assured that " truth "
won't " be beaten " in a fair " fight ".[2] Is this an echo
of an infantile struggle against the disciplining parents ?
At least that was the first sort of struggle which the child
knew.[3]

One of the forms most usually assumed by the argument against censorship of opinion, is a boast that it

[1] The last two paragraphs are by Moyle (G. W.), in *Los Angeles
Record*, May 23rd, 1923. This utterance was prompted by the events
in Los Angeles Harbour, to which I refer presently.
[2] " Magna est veritas et praevalebit."
[3] Though breaking wind is forbidden to the child, yet he jealously
notes that the father (as psycho-analytic writers have pointed out) is
more free than the women members of the household in passing flatus,
which indeed becomes a symbol of his potency—*vide* Jones's patient,
who had a recurring dream on the greatness of God's works as displayed in thunder storms which burst open the back doors.
Jones (E.), " A Case of Obsessional Neurosis ", *Jahrbach der Psycho-
analyse*, bd. V. Republ. in his *Papers on Psycho-Analysis* (London,
1923), p. 538. Flügel tells me that the entire life of a patient of his
was determined by his reactions as a child to the freedom with which
his father passed flatus.

doesn't castrate the sons at all.   They become, if anything, more potent than before.

" Ideas are always liveliest when attempts are made to
suppress them. The very worst way to suppress an idea
is to attempt to suppress it, and if it is false it does not need
to be suppressed, it will suppress itself." (Horace Traubel).
" Men are imprisoned, their words spread wider for that
fact. The mere publication in a newspaper of the statement of a leading radical—' I am for the people, and the
government is for the profiteers '—was considered so dangerous to the morale of soldiers who might read it that she was
sentenced to ten years in prison, yet her words were repeated by every important newspaper in the country during
the trial."[1]

We shall generally find that those who figure as rebels
in various other movements, economic, political, etc.,
are in favour of freedom of speech.   An exception must
be made in the case of the communists.   The sponsors
of the Workers' Education Associations in Britain and
America are keen to seize upon evidences that the
existing system of schools and universities inculcates
pro-capitalistic ideas in the youth of the land, and claim
themselves to be fair.   But a communist magazine
laments that in ordinary colleges,

" The teaching claims to be, and usually is, impartial."[2]

whereas the horde-brothers ought to abet their own
collective potency :

" The function of a Labour College should be the diffusion
of ideas most likely to assist the Labour Movement."[3]

[1] Chafee (Prof. Z.), *Propaganda and Conscription in the Next War.*
New York, 1925.
[2] " That is, it is an attempt to dissuade working men from taking
an active part in the class war."
The juxtaposition of this and the preceding phrases indicates an
ambivalent attitude.   From a brochure : *The Industrial Peace*, quoted
by *The Plebs*, Oxford, May, 1918, vol. X, no. 4, p. 118.
[3] *The Plebs*, Oxford, March, 1909, vol. I, no. 2, p. 27.

with the aim of eventually usurping the Old Man's place.

"Labour the slave, Labour the rebel, must become Labour the ruler."[1]

Catastrophic Reform

In many phantasies of rescuing society from its oppressors, the work is to be done by a single bold stroke —the assassination, say, of a tyrant, or the plan of " the general strike "—a fact which leads to the view that the killing or castration of the father is what the repressed complex really aims at. For the teaching of history is abundant as to the futility of such methods in the political world.

In this connection Bertrand Russell has made the enlightening observation that :

"a large proportion of revolutionary leaders have had ideas extremely like Shelley's. They have thought that misery and cruelty and degradation were due to tyrants, or priests, or capitalists, or Germans, and that if these sources of evil were overthrown there would be a general change of heart and we should all live happy ever after. Holding these beliefs, they have been willing to wage a ' war to end war '. Comparatively fortunate were those who suffered defeat or death ; those who had the misfortune to emerge victorious were reduced to cynicism and despair by the failure of all their glowing hopes. The ultimate source of these hopes," [Russell concludes], " was the Christian doctrine of catastrophic conversion as the road to salvation."[2]

But it would surely be more accurate to say that all these hopes were alike the outcome of what must come far earlier than any of them in every individual's life, namely the repressed childhood belief in murder or castration of the father as the road to the mother.

---

[1] *The Plebs.* Oxford, February, 1909, vol. I, no. [1], p 9.
[2] Russell (B.), " Salvation ; Individual and Social ", in *What I Believe* (London, 1925), p. 71.

HUMANITARIAN TYPE

The castrating and killing phantasies, as we shall find, enter into the task of the penal reformer, and of those who would mitigate animal cruelty or warfare.

Penal Reform

Crime, apparently, is often an expression of defiance against the state conceived of as the commanding parent. This receives confirmation from the irrationality of criminals, who, after repeated proofs of the unprofitableness of their career, return to the old ways as often as released from punishment.[1]

The studies of Burt on the sources of crime are valuable testimony as to its close connection with unresolved personal conflicts.[2]

Some years ago, the present writer, during the tedium of a brief incarceration as a political prisoner had opportunity for long talks with several professional criminals. He was much struck by the attitude of resignation to fate which some of them evinced. These felt it was entirely hopeless to plan for a future any different from what their past had been ; temptation was sure to come again, and something within would compel them to yield. Indeed, of the one per cent. or so of the popula-

---

[1] Consider this as a case :—

"A pretty Irish servant girl listened with an air of boredom to the tale of her remarkable career told to Hove magistrates yesterday.

"Aged 19, she had been twice convicted for being drunk and disorderly, and had served months hard labour for wandering abroad. She had been in seven convents, said her mother. From one she ran away, and the authorities at the other six had sent her away because of her violent temper.

"She was now charged on remand with wandering abroad, without visible means of subsistence.

"'I don't want her to go to prison again,' said her mother, 'it doesn't seem to do her any good '." *Daily Herald*, London, January 14th, 1924.

[2] Burt (Cyril), *The Young Delinquent*, pp. 566-7.

tion which forms the criminal class, a surprisingly large number are recidivists.

A consciousness of these same criminal impulses in themselves give some other persons, who know how to deal with them more rationally, their sympathy with the unfortunates in prisons. The reader will recall the story of Bunyan, who, seeing a felon led away to be hanged, exclaimed, " There, but for the grace of God, goes John Bunyan ! "

Fortunately, for the peace of society, the Œdipus complex does not work wholly for the increase of crime. For, as we have already seen, the prototype of criminals is the child's own father, the assumed assaulter of his mother. On this account, a portion of the Œdipus complex is enlisted against the criminal.

Indeed, this is one obstacle which is met with by humane reformers of our criminal code. They find that the criminal has become a convenient scapegoat on which society unloads much father-hatred even against society's own demonstrated advantages and interest. Says " Mr Dooley " :

" I don't believe in capital punishment, Hinnisay, but 'twill never be abolished while th' people injie it so much."[1]

Animal Welfare. Pacifism

Onto dumb animals, as well as against human beings, there may well be directed some of the father-hatred. This would account for a part of the public's heartlessness toward them—the over-burdening, trapping, baiting, and hunting them which has only been a little mitigated in a few Buddhist and Christian lands.[1]

By a somewhat different mechanism to that which made the sons regard the criminal as a hated father, they tend to regard the war profiteers as such. There are two tangible possessions for which the father is

[1] " Mr Dooley," quoted by Sprading (C. T.), *Liberty and the Great Libertarians* (Los Angeles, 1913), p. 34.

especially envied by the son. The one which earliest
excites jealousy is, as so many psycho-analysts have
found, the paternal phallus, which is so much larger
than the son's own. The other is, the father's wealth.

Both of these tangible things the son intuitively or
otherwise (the reader will recall our reference to Dr
Melanie Klein's analyses of children) associates with
the father's pre-eminent status in the family, and with
that attribute which we may vaguely call power. Phallus
or property, that is to say, may either one be regarded
as the father's sword by the power of which he mounts
guard over the beloved mother and fends off the son
from peaceful possession of her. Or either may be
regarded as *par excellence* the father's organ of potency.

Interesting, therefore, as an outgrowth of a suspicion
that the father's desires, if they do not actually instigate
the *wars* to which the sons have to march to their death
(a suspicion we shall discuss in a later chapter)[1] is a
proposal to castrate the fathers by cutting off their
organ of potency, property, whenever they send the sons
to be slaughtered.

> " To the end that war may be made as repellent to all
> classes as it is to those who must fight, the *Christian Science
> Monitor* has proposed an amendment to the Constitution
> of the United States, expressed in substance as follows :—
> " ' in the event of a declaration of war, the property,
> equally with the persons, lives and liberties of all citizens,
> shall be subject to conscription for the defence of the nation,
> and it shall be the duty of the President to propose, and of
> the Congress to enact, the legislation necessary to give
> effect to this amendment.' "[2]

[1] p. 192, below.
[2] As representing the property-monopolizing fathers, the senior
generation generally is in favour of whatever steps the protection of the
property-institution may require. At the time that the United States
was debating the question of greater military preparedness in case she
should be dragged into the Great War, the Business Mens' League
made an appeal based on the consideration that a more militarised
community would better subserve the propertied and employing
interests :—
" Let us have no more class legislation or we will have it repealed
with bayonets. . . .

RELIGIO-THERAPEUTIC TYPE

In primitive magic, we treat the thing's representative
as we should like to treat the thing represented.

" Business men should be sensible of the advantages . . . of greater
discipline . . . of the work people.

" In the general apprehension for greater preparedness to cope with
foreign nations, it is believed that a necessity fully as grave is being
overlooked, or at least greatly minimised ; that is the need for an
adequate military establishment to act as a civil police force. . . .

" In the hearings before the Industrial Relations Commission at
Seattle, a representative business man, Mr J. V. Paterson, addressing
the labour members on the commission with great courage, stated :
' We will fight you. We will rise with a counter revolution—we certainly have the power. We will destroy you. Let us have no more
class legislation, or we will have to repeal it with bayonets ; we will do
it, no doubt about that.'

" Due to lack of sufficient militia, business men in the United States
have frequently been placed under the undue burden of having to engage
for the services of men recruited privately and to have them com-
missioned as deputies by the civil authorities. In the nature of things,
these private forces are without efficient military training, as at Youngs-
town, Ohio, in Pennsylvania and elsewhere. In the single month of
October, in 1913, the meagre military forces of four separate states
were required in the field against labour, in Calumet, Michigan, in
Indianapolis, and in Colorado and West Virginia.

" . . . It must be remembered that the Federal troops were required
to suppress the strike of the American Railway Union. . . .

" In this entire matter business men should be sensible of the advantages to be had from military training in point of greater discipline
. . . of the work people for their own ordinary civil employment.
Every employee returning from training camp or militia drill will
forthwith show himself more obedient and faithful, and the trouble-
maker will disappear." *Announcement of the Pacific Coast Business
Men's* preparedness league.

" At the 33rd annual convention of the International Association of
Chiefs of Police, held in Chicago, July 19th to 22nd, 1926, a great point
was made of utilizing the developments of chemical warfare for ' dis-
persing strike meetings, making labour and other halls uninhabitable ',
etc.

" Thus the Lake Erie Chemical Co., of Cleveland, urges [the use of]
its Dispers-X irritating gas and smoke against ' strike mobs containing
women and children '. It recommends its Blind-X Riot gun as an
' ideal weapon for defending industrial plants ', etc. It offers its
Exile-X chemical to make ' sure that the same den will not be used for
meeting or living quarters for a long time, probably one month '.

" This company uses an ex-army officer to train state constabularies
and police forces in the use of the gases. . . .

" The exhibitor of another gas concern, the Federal Laboratories,
Inc. of Pittsburg, mentioned with pride the use of tear bombs against
the textile strikers of Passaic. ' Why, you can knock out a whole
family, from father to baby, with one of our gas grenades,' he said,
' then walk in and grab the man and let the rest recover at leisure '."
American Appeal, Chicago, August 7th, 1921.

So one may symbolically deny the father any existence by denying existence to his heavenly prototype. Agnosticism, atheism, materialism and rationalism probably owe a great debt to this mechanism of motivation. One bit of evidence for this statement is found in the close correlation between the beliefs mentioned and such movements of revolt against the old (=fathers') order as are anarchism, communism, guildism, socialism, and syndicalism. Particularly true is this of the founders of these movements, and of the group who become attracted to them before they have become at all respectable. But the phantasy of doing away with the father enters into the psychology both of unbelievers and of believers.

Unbelievers

Marx and Hyndman may serve as illustrations, and we have also Jeremy Bentham as an excellent example, of the relationship between atheism and father-hatred. We have already seen how bitterly Bentham lampooned his father's profession, etc. This same revolting son admitted consistently enough :

" To the Almighty, I must confess I know not how to render myself anything better than an ' unprofitable servant ' : as to what concerns my fellow man, I am not without hope."[1]

His biographer, Bowring, records a confession which connects Bentham's irreligion with his youthful father-relationship in a very direct way :

" One of my tribulations at this time used to be learning church collects. They used to give me the colic, but my father insisted on my getting them by heart."[2]

An absolute denial of the existence of the father is

[1] Bentham (J.), *Jeremy Bentham to Citizens of the United States*, " Letter VIII ", 1817.
[2] Bowring (J.), *Works of Jeremy Bentham*.

paramount to banishing him or putting him out of the
way ; which is what children mean by killing.

Moreover, the fact that a majority of the older generation profess adherence to the doctrines of the Church,
connects adherence to these doctrines with the father-
loving attitude, and connects defection from them with
the father-despising one.   In an age like the present one,
in which the rebellious spirit is uppermost, independence
of belief becomes more fashionable than conformity
to the group, that is to say, to the father.   The two
attitudes are mutually inconsistent.[1]

The reader will find that the rule we have enunciated
holds true in a striking degree in the case of all those
men whom we have had cause to mention in this thesis
who are atheists and about whom adequate information
is readily obtainable.   Those whom I am listing here-
with are not selected for the sake of proving the point.
I am simply putting down in chronological order those
atheists about whom I incidentally obtained biographical
data in connection with their relationship to a completely different movement, namely, socialism ; i.e.
the selection is, for the purpose in hand, a random one.

First, of course, comes Karl Marx.   The reader will
recall enough of what has been said of him to realize
that if Marx became a rationalist, it was certainly not
through predominance in his make up of the reflective
over the emotional tendencies.   He regularly acted less
like one who has come to a conclusion upon some question through the process of rational thought, than like a

---

[1] " One cannot agree with a solid group of people . . . and preserve
independent judgment. . . .
" The present-day decay of the Church is probably thus to be explained.   Right to individual opinion and interpretation is being
granted more and more.   If faith becomes individual, there is no need
for communal exercise of the rites that go with faith.   Religious organ-
isation is, and must be, founded on dogma and intolerance.   As the
latter are no longer popular, social caste has largely been substituted
for community of faith as the cement of Church organisations.   Since
castes have other means of expressing their cohesion, the Churches
have not gained by this change of motifs."   MacCurdy, *Dynamic
Psychology* (London), p. 325, footnote.

man who finds in certain lines of conduct an expression for an old deep smouldering hatred for he knows not whom. Whatever represents authority and compulsion stirs up this old hate ; certain individual men arouse it too.

Few readers will need to have it pointed out to them that suspicion in such a case naturally falls upon the relationship between our hero and his father. If the usual Œdipus complex had arisen between Marx senior and the son who was destined to be the founder of modern socialism, the facts of that son's life are strictly *en regle*.

The father, as we know, was a Prussian official, a conservative, and (notwithstanding that he introduced his son to anti-theological authors) a religious man, sincerely converted from Judaism to Christianity.[1]

In the case of William Morris,[2] the most direct cause of apostacy was hatred of his clerical schoolmasters, but the schoolmaster is regularly a father-surrogate. One of his biographers relates that :

> " The stress of the officialism that bore upon him in his public school career, previously to which he had been sent to Forest School, in his native place . . . left a less agreeable, if not less enduring, impression. ' I was educated at Marlborough under clerical masters, and I naturally rebelled against them '."

Let us consider next, the late H. M. Hyndman, of whom Bernard Shaw, speaking from intimate acquaint-

[1] " The father was a converted Jew, the son was an ardently atheistic materialist ; but the father was also a curious blend of Prussian patriot and admirer of the humane scepticism of Voltaire." Salter (F. R.), *Karl Marx and Modern Socialism* (London, 1921), p. 6.
" When he was six years old, the family was converted to Christianity . . . as a result of that romantic idealising of Christianity of which Chateaubriand was the most famous representative. . . . To the end of his life he remained something of an anti-semite ; but this does not seem traceable to any emotion of apostacy." Laski (N. J.), *Karl Marx* (London, 1922).
[2] " William Morris, the eldest of five sons, was destined for the church, and for that reason was entered, at the age of fourteen, at Marlboro' College, there to be educated under clerical masters." Sticknew (G.), *William Morris*, p. 3.

ance, said that he " took the very definite anti-religious attitude of the mid-nineteenth century ".[1]

We find Hyndman himself admitting this attitude, and, in the same paragraph, his sharp divergence on such matters from his hated father—all true to the form of the Œdipus complex :

> " I was born of strictly religious parents, indeed exceedingly devout. I was brought up in an atmosphere of the sincerest devotion, and was surrounded by prayer and praise to God and His Christ. Moreover, I believe in my way I am not devoid of religious feeling of a kind. Yet, somehow, even my mother, who was greatly disturbed at this peculiarity, was quite unable to get me to pray . . . I have never been able to accept the view that appeals to a personal deity could be anything more than a personal gratification of individual sentiments. My brothers and sisters . . . by no means shared my opinions on these points. They were true believers of a very ardent type, and conservatives in politics as well."[2]

Believers

But it is time we turned from examination of non-believers to their opposites, who manifest faith in excess.

When a New Thought leader carries the doctrine of cheerfulness, as does Trine in some doggerel verses of his, to the point of advising friends not to lament those who have died, on the score that their once-loved forms were " not worth a single tear ",[3] he evinces abnormally

---

[1] Conversation with the writer, November 27th, 1924. And Mrs Hyndman wrote : " As a freethinker, Hyndman was more of a definite materialist than an agnostic, a man of the sixtys rather than of the nineties. His first instinct was to say, ' There is nothing ', rather than, ' I do not know '. . . . When he was young a singularly ugly and unreasonable form of theology had been presented to him with all the definiteness and authority of a scientific formula." Hyndman (R. T.), *Last Years of H. M. Hyndman* (London, 1923), p. 38.

[2] Hyndman (H. M.), *Record of an Adventurous Life* (London, 1911), p. 8

[3] " To those less strong he, the New Thought, adherent can say :—
" ' Loving friends ! be wise and dry
Straightway every weeping eye ;
What you left upon the bier
Is not worth a single tear.' "
Trine (R. W.), *In Tune with the Infinite* (London, 1923), p. 115.

calloused feelings. Whence may such an inhibition of natural sentiments as is implied by ability to take this cold philosophic outlook, be derived ? Inhibitions are due to counter tendencies ; therefore, Trine would appear to betray that he has felt repressed hatred toward someone whom he either " left upon the bier ", or dreamed of so leaving.

Baudoin, whose name is so closely associated with that of Coué, gives us a very frank picture of himself as a child indulging in thinly disguised death-wishes against his parents. These wishes are, moreover, combined with thoughts about some secret knowledge of which the parents are the happy possessors. In a certain childhood scene the little boy, left behind in a garden, reflects :

> " My father and mother must be extremely good to be able to walk about and talk so quietly amidst things incomprehensible to me ; yes, indeed, what troubled me must be perfectly clear to them ; never should I dare confess that they amazed me, for then should I appear to them stupid and very strange to myself. No one ever told me to be thus amazed . . . And I repeated aloud the words ' almost dead ', as I stared at the back of the pink coat . . .
> " I felt a certain delight in dwelling upon this idea : ' almost dead '." [1]

Now to sum up the foregoing chapter : Castration has been attempted symbolically by censorship, catastrophic revolutions, and conscription of property. Men also have tried to do away with the father by doing away with criminals, the state, or God.

---

[1] Baudoin (Ch.), *Birth of Psyche*, transl. Rothwell (London, 1923), p. 52.

CHAPTER V

AMBIVALENCE; AND THE GOD COMPLEX

INTRODUCTORY REMARKS

AMBIVALENCE is a term invented by Bleuler[1] for the phenomena first called by Stekel *bipolarity*, namely the fact that one may simultaneously feel both affection and dislike for the same person. Freud points out that such a condition is more usual in neurotic than in normal persons[2]. Nevertheless this constellation does often occur in the normal, as he illustrates in a footnote by a quotation from the *symposium* in which Alcibiades says of Socrates:

"Many a time have I wished that he were dead, and yet I know that I should be much more sorry than glad if he were to die; so that I am at my wits' end."[3]

Elsewhere[4] Freud shows how positive and negative aspects of an instinct may successively be put forth, and how both of these aspects may go on existing in the unconscious.

Now, both of these developments may have been going on simultaneously. Moreover, says Freud, the individual may retain elements of the earlier stages of development of the impulse in question, right alongside of later stages of its development. Freud uses here the simile of successive lava flows on the flank of a volcano; recent layers of lava may lie in contact with very ancient and quite differently composed layers, although they have all issued from the same crater. Freud concludes with the statement:

[1] Bleuler, E.: Lecture "Ambivalence," in Berne, 1910, abstracted in *Zeutrablatt für Psycho-Analyse*, Bd. I, S. 266. Also article "Dementia Praecox oder Gruppe der Schizophrenien" in Aschaffenburg: *Handbuch der Psychiatrie*, 1911.
[2] Freud, S.: *Collected Papers*, London, 1924, vol. II, p. 320.
[3] Jowett's Translation. See Freud (S.), *idem*, vol. III, p. 375.
[4] Freud, S., *idem*, vol. IV, pp. 72-74.

"The fact that, at a later period of development, the instinct in its primary form may be observed side by side with its (passive) opposite deserves to be distinguished by the . . . name . . . ambivalence."[1]

Let me venture myself to give an illustration from actual life, of a conflict arising from this very instinct of scoptophilia-exhibitionism. A person known to me had sublimated his impulse *to look at* things (originally, at the penis) through various stages into an interest in the science of psychology. The impulse to be (originally to have his penis) looked at remained at a cruder level, having only reached the stage where it prompted him to be sensationally conspicuous. Naturally these two lines of development greatly interfered with one another. For at the very time when the subject's scientific interests urged him to do careful work and to seek association with other psychologists in their societies, etc., his exhibitionism betrayed him into premature publication of half-verified conclusions, or it manouvered him into notoriety that came near costing him some coveted society memberships.

Of course, we are not concerned in the present paper with scoptophilia nor exhibitionism. These were referred to merely to illustrate the working of ambivalence. For I have thought it would be fitting to conclude this Part I of my thesis, which has dealt with mechanisms opposed to the father, and to proceed to Part II, which will deal with those working in his favour, with a chapter on ambivalence. This will mark a kind of halfway position of mixed motivation.

Among these father-mechanisms, ambivalent as regards the father, is one of such surpassing importance as to merit a few words of special explanation. I refer to the *God complex*, which prompts to a mode of behaviour and reasoning that would only be justifiable if the subject were God.

Since *God* equals father *magnified*, one may in phantasy achieve the childish desire to be the equal or

[1] *Idem*, p. 74.

superior of one's father, by picturing one's self as god-like. That this phantasy is actually and frequently indulged in must be clear to those who have read Jones' notable essay on the " God Complex ".[1]

The belief in question is not only an expression of enormous narcissism, but a form of relegation of the father to a subordinate position and of usurpation of his privileges, such as jealous sons desire. While Narcissism is undoubtedly the main motive in this complex, we should not forget that (a) the super-ego is developed out of the father-image ; (b) the figure of God is similarly derived ; and (c) the belief that one is God clearly subserves a desire to equal through identity, if not to surpass, the father, the boy's earliest rival.

Of this God-complex, perhaps the most outstanding sub-trait is what Freud quotes a neurotic, Schreber, naming *the omnipotence of thought*. By this he meant a conviction that by merely thinking a thing to be so, it was made to be so. This is partly a development of that narcissism which likes to imagine that the universe turns upon ourselves as pivot. But it would appear also or chiefly to be derived, according to Jones, from the association between *thought* and *paternal flatus*,[2] which, in its turn, is a symbol for the father's potency. Thought is, moreover, so closely connected with various such forms of its expression as gestures, cries and speech, that it must itself become associated with some of the efficacy an infant finds these gestures, etc., to possess, towards getting his wants satisfied.

ECONOMICO POLITICAL TYPE

Among the economic movements of our day which are notably ambivalent in their attitude toward the father are co-operativism, communism and socialism.

---

[1] Jones (E.), " The God Complex ", in his *Essays in Applied Psycho-Analysis* (London, 1923), pp. 204 ff.

[2] Jones (E.), " The Holy Ghost ", in his *Essays in Applied Psycho-Analysis* (London, 1923).

H

Co-operation

I have thus far not mentioned an extremely important movement of our day, that of Co-operativism. It is, however, a very appropriate one to consider under the caption of ambivalence, because the middle position which it occupies as between capitalism and socialism makes it relatively to the one a rebel-son-movement, so to speak, while relatively to the other it appears as a father movement.

As the ancient Egyptians could regard the sun (especially when setting) as the father, Osiris, and yet see in the same sun (especially when rising) Ra, the hero-son, so the adherents of other progressive movements sometimes look upon the co-operators as conservatives, sometimes as radicals.

Here, for instance, is the utterance of a socialist who hates the co-operativists as submissive sons who side with the father ; he says :

"the trade co-operator canonizes the burgeois virtues, but socialist vices, of ' overwork ' and ' thrift '."[1]

To the working-man, the bourgeois is a father-figure on account of his greater wealth, social prestige, education and position as potential employer. In . this passage we have again that childish protest against industry and thrift, which already has been touched on.

The co-operative movement applies on the one hand, the conservative principle of saving, and even leans so far " to the right " as to excite the disgust of many of the more extreme revolutionists. " Why do you always crab at the co-operatives ? " H. M. Hyndman was asked by his wife. " Because ", he replied in effect, our English co-operatives do not, like the Belgians and others, invest their earnings in social halls and educational and other efforts toward a larger communal life for their members, but are concerned only with petty dividends.

[1] Bax (Belfort), *Religion of Socialism*, p. 94.   Quoted in *Anti-Socialist Union Speakers' Handbook*, pp. 252-3.

We may surmise that the friction which the British co-operatives have, of late years, experienced with their employees, may have represented in part the fact that their relationship reawakened the old quarrel of father and sons. Less than a year ago, England echoed with the cry, raised by a Tory, but repeated by extreme left wingers, that in the co-operatives, Britain had a million small capitalists.

On the other hand, since co-operativism represents a breaking down of the tendency towards increasing division of the population into a few possessors of enormous wealth and a dispossessed proletariat, it has certain elements of appeal to the sons.

An outsider may judge a person or a movement better than an insider can. Co-operativism at any rate has managed to stir the ire of the conservative element. In the United States, especially, where the movement still is just winning its foothold, the grossest misrepresentation of its aims, and most untruthful allegations against its success, not to speak of insinuations against the honesty of its leaders and morality of its followers, are usual.

Strangely enough, it is in a very different camp from that of the co-operatives that we find another example of a movement which is highly ambivalent. I refer to Bolshevism. It is the most left-wing of economico-political movements to-day, unless we accept anarchism. Yet Eder[1] maintains that what has given Bolshevism more cohesion than other revolutionary movements has been its father veneration, as exemplified in the omnipresent busts of Marx.

Communism

Bolshevism is coloured through and through with the personality of Lenin, who established it in Russia. One commonly thinks of this great figure as the most rebellious of rebel sons. But Lenin was also the *father* of the new revolutionary regime, and *head* of the new state. In this

[1] Eder (M. D.), " Psycho-Analysis and Politics ", in *Social Aspects of Psycho-Analysis*, ed. by E. Jones (London, 1923).

capacity, his Œdipus Complex found quite an opposite expression. Consider, in evidence, his argument about

" Forced syndicalisation—that is, forced fusion into unions under the control of the state. This is what capitalism has prepared for us. This is what the Banker State has realised in Germany. This is what will be completely realisable in Russia by the Soviets, by the dictatorship of the proletariat. This is what the state-apparatus, universal, newest and non-bureaucratic, will give us."[1]

The communist party, as a whole, and in various countries, has shown the same tendency as its heroic leader, to this ambivalence of attitude. In Russia, the Bolsheviks got their name through being the majority section of the socialist party—in other words, the father-element within a rebellious son-movement. Rightly or wrongly, a reputation for double dealing dogs all their attempts to open up commercial relations with other countries.

In the United States at any meeting at which miscellaneous rebellious movements are represented—· Anarchist, Socialist, I.W.W., Workers' Party, Communist, etc.—all remain brothers to at least the extent of tolerating one another's criticisms, until someone criticizes communism. The communists present thereupon break up the meeting.[2]

The ambivalence of attitude to which I refer is observable in many of the notes sent out from Moscow to the communist parties of other countries. Towards the capitalists, the communists are urged to be rebellious

---

[1] Ulianov (V. : Lenin, N.), *Will the Bolsheviks Maintain Power ?* (London, 1922), p. 53.

[2] A notable example of this conduct occurred in New York in the Spring of 1925, at a meeting held under the auspices of the Civil Liberties' Union, on behalf of political and industrial prisoners throughout the world. All at first went well, and the fact that men were still held in jail in the States of the U.S., and elsewhere because of pacifist, industrial or political activities, was condemned. Then a speaker mentioned that another country which held such prisoners was Russia. At once the pro-father complexes of the communists responded ; there was a riot,

sons, but toward other left wing parties they are to be stern fathers if the communists themselves are in power, but rebellious sons still if the others come into office. I wish now to speak of a somewhat different matter. I may begin by saying that impulsions which have their true origin within oneself, are often *projected* on to outside parties. A familiar example of this is that of paranoiacs who project their own morbidly accusing consciences on to other persons (persecution mania). Another example is found in absurdedly jealous persons, whose jealousy is really attributing to the wife (or husband) desires felt by the jealous mate himself. In the following letter from Lenin, note how the accusation of ambivalence (" treacherous natures ") is projected on to the other parties (such epithets are commonplaces in present-day Russian political language).

"In Britain . . . we must first help Henderson and Snowden to defeat Lloyd George and Churchill . . . . Secondly, we must help the majority of the working-class to convince themselves of the utter worthlessness of the Hendersons and Snowdens, of their petty bourgeois and treacherous natures, of the inevitability of their bankruptcy."[1]

The ambivalent attitude of the Bolsheviks towards other working-class movements has inspired a like ambivalent[2] attitude in return on the part of the latter. In recent years this has been especially noticeable in England.

[1] Lenin (N.), *Collected Works*, Russian ed., vol. XVII, p. 165. Excerpted by Lepeshinsky (A.), *Lenin and Britain* (London), p. 81.

[2] The mechanism can be elucidated by reference to its *modus operandi* in dreams.

"Conceptions which stand in opposition to one another are preferably expressed in dreams by the same element. Eminent philologists maintain that the oldest language used the same word for expressing quite general antithesis. . . . In C. Abel's essay, ' Uber den Gegensinn der Urwörter ', (1884), the following examples of such words in English are given : ' gleam—gloom ' ; ' to lock—loch ' ; ' down—The Downs ' ; ' to stop—to stop '. . . . See also Freud, ' Ueber den Gegensinn der Urwörter ' : *Jahrbuch fur Psychoanalytische Forschimgen*, Band u, part 1, p. 179." Freud (S.), *On Dreams*, transl. Eder (London), pp. 59-60.

Socialism

In this country the labour party has, on the one hand, stood for closer relationship with Russia, while, on the other, it declined to admit communists to its membership. On the one hand, the socialists have recognized the opposition between their constitutionalist policy, and the violent policy of communism ; on the other, they have flirted with the latter movement. This they have done notwithstanding that the flirtation has cost them dear, by providing a weapon for enemies who represent both factions as being " tarred with the same brush ".

Where such self-injuring tactics are used, an observer is bound to attribute them to some repressed factor. This may consist in a Hamlet-like[1] hesitation (ambivalence) in attacking those who by overthrowing Tzardom and capitalism in Russia (murder of the royal father) have laid low a figure whom the labour party themselves hated. It seems certainly to represent some impulse at self thwarting, similar to that in Freud's

> " Report of a young mechanical engineer, which gives some insight into the mechanism of damaging things. He and several others had involuntarily undertaken some tests which demanded more of their time than anticipated, so that a friend one day jokingly said, ' Let us hope that the machine will refuse to work, so that we can . . . go home earlier '."

[1] See Freud's and Jones' studies of Hamlet. That Shakespeare-Hamlet felt the heavy hand of the fathers as a social as well as a personal phenomenon is indicated in the well-known lines about

> " The whips and scorns of time,
> The oppressor's wrong, the proud man's contumely.
> The insolence of office, and the spurns
> That patient merit of the unworthy takes."

In *King Lear*, also, Shakespeare says :—
> " Take physic, pomp ;
> Expose thyself to feel what wretches feel.
> That thou mayest shake the superflux to them
> And show the heavens more just."

F. chanced to be assigned the duty of opening the pressure valve. The leader of the experiment

> " called a ' Stop ' when the maximum pressure was reached. At this command F. grasped the valve and turned it with all his force, to the left hand (all valves . . . are closed to the right). This caused a sudden full pressure . . . and as there was no outlet, the connecting pipe burst. This was . . . enough to force us to stop our work . . . and go home."[1]

Returning now to the subject we were discussing, we need not go to the communists for giving a social ideal such expression as is calculated to arouse more hearers to oppose it than to become adherents. Beside its half-heartedness in repudiating the violence and dictatorship of communistic tactics, socialism has suffered through its individual exponents who directly connected it with other ideals not likely to be popular. It has been well said that what chiefly hinders the success of any movement is not anything done by its opponents, but the acts and words of unwisely zealous friends.

Socialism would to-day be nearer its goal if half of its zealots had never expressed themselves. It is unfair to a movement to condemn it on the score of the most extreme utterances of which any adherent has been guilty publicly or privately ; just as it would be to condemn, say, Great Britain, because of a speech made by one of her officials. Extreme opinions balance each other ; we must base criticism on official party documents. Nevertheless opponents will not make such allowances ; and utterances like the above turn powerful forces against the cause for which they were spoken. They have helped to enlist the father-hating complex against, instead of for, the proposed revolution by making it appear as a mere substitution of a severer father for a milder one. The very quotation I have taken is cited

[1] Freud (S.), *Psychopathology of Everyday Life*, transl. Brill (London, 1922), pp. 190-1.

as a warning to the public, in the *Anti-Socialist Speakers'
Handbook*. The reader will also recall that Herbert
Spencer, prior to his own conversion to a qualified
socialism, called it " the coming slavery ".

It is difficult to determine the point of division between
fear of a movement because it represents to the person
fearing a tightening of father-like oppression, and fear
of it rather because one identifies oneself with the father
and looks on the movement as a castration threat
against him by the sons. In the passages below, these
two attitudes are condensed. The writers are partly
sons rebelling against despotism and tyranny and the
mandate that children should be seen and not heard.
But yet that which they want heard is, not sons' irrever-
ent voices, but that of the father (religion). The first
writer, a Dr Schäffle, does

> " not believe that social democracy would permit freedom
> to the religious life. It would of necessity be far more
> intolerant than the existing state."[1]

The second writer enlarges on the same sentiment. The
paternal state, he feels, would forbid the sons to sow
their *seed* :

> " Freedom of thought would perish under socialism . . .
> Thoughts are the seeds of mighty movements, and is it
> likely that the socialist state would encourage that which
> might very easily end in its overthrow and destruction ?
> . . . Least of all, would socialism encourage religious free-
> dom, because religion has ever been the most potent instru-
> ment of revolution, and socialism, though it would usurp
> itself by means of revolution, would seek to maintain its
> power by despotism and tyranny."[2]

We have seen that in the case of Karl Marx, a strong
antagonism evidently existed towards his father. The
trait was closely blended, in Marx's case, with a most
inordinate egotism, bordering on the god-complex, or

---

[1] Schäffle (Dr.), *Impossibility of Social Democracy*, p. 167. Quoted
by *Anti-Socialist Speakers' Handbook*, p. 220.
[2] *Anti-Socialist Speakers' Handbook* (London, 1911), p. 220.

belief that one is God. Both this trait and the rever-
berations of this boyhood antagonism appear in the fact
that through his life

> " Marx never welcomed opposition or rivalry ; and he
> was too prone to assume that a doubt of his rightness was
> justification for a doubt also of his opponent's integrity."[1]

Marx's intense insistence that circumstances determine
men, and that we must never blame the individual, but
only the institutions which created and schooled him,
i.e. fathered him, was perhaps a way of saying " Everything is father's fault ", or " See what a mess father
makes of the world ! " The people and institutions he
was opposed to, all became (to judge by his vindictive
fury) father types. In addition, it is possible that the
reiteration that what counted in the world was circumstances and not personalities, was a defence mechanism.
By it Marx saved his own self esteem from realizing the
fact, so patent to all but himself, that his own life was
really determined altogether too much by personalities—
the echoes of one personality (his father's) in particular.
This constituted probably his gravest defect of character,
and raised up innumerable enemies against him and
consequently against the movement he so largely
moulded.

> " The contempt which he showered so lavishly on most
> of his contemporaries came from a complete failure to under-

---

[1] " Impatient of difference, as with Proudhon and Bakunin, contemptuous, as his correspondence with Engels shows, of all who did
not think exactly in his fashion, he never learned the essential art of
colleagueship. He was too prone to regard a hostile view as a proof
of moral crime. He had not a little of that zest for priority he was so
unwilling to recognize in the discoveries of others. He was rarely
generous in his recognition of intellectual stimulus. With Marx, to
enter a movement was to dominate it ; and he was incapable of taking
the second place. ' Hatred ', wrote Mazzini of him, ' outweighs love in
his heart, which is not right even if the hatred may in itself have foundation '.
" There is something unhealthy in the venom with which he assails
early friends like Bruno Bauer, or not less ardent seekers after light
like Proudhon. His accusations against Proudhon, even when the
temptation . . . to destroy is remembered, are singularly ungenerous."
Laski (H. J.), *Karl Marx* (London), pp. 25-6.

stand or make any allowances for any standpoint other than his own . . . There was a real weakness in the narrowness of outlook, and, like Carlyle, Marx belongs to the prophet tribe rather than to the scientists ; he delivered oracles, he did not examine evidences. This may appear a ridiculous criticism in view of his most painstaking and careful analysis of the capitalist system of production, but . . . the reasoning faculties are only allowed to begin at a certain point."[1]

To leave Marx and to generalize a bit, one reason that our politics are so confused and ineffective is that they are determined by ambivalent attitudes on our part. Our jealousy of the father makes us avow ourselves democrats ; but in practice, our democratic governmental forms are negated by concessions to the father as priest, official and proprietor.

In an article in *Psyche and Eros,* Theodore Schroeder expounds at length the view that our concessions to democracy are a mere lip-service, a legal fiction, and that :

" The American Revolution was fought to establish a democratic fiction in place of a theocratic fiction . . . "

But under either outward form, the right of the fathers to exploit the sons economically has always been recognized. Indeed, the people connive at the deportation of those

" Whose chief offence may be no more than a demand that we live up to our fiction . . .
" Because mankind has been so largely functioning on the level of this conflict we have sought to reform through the adoption of a new fiction, a new law, or a new theory of government. Inevitably, therefore, our past revolutions have been practical failures when judged from the standpoint of the objective reality of their achievement. Subjectively they supplied a great satisfaction. We, the revolutionists and their successors, have shown our relative omnipotence by overthrowing the Almighty ones who had previously dominated in the name of God.

[1] Salter (F. R.), *Karl Marx and Modern Socialism* (London, 1921), p. 12.

" The chairman of the Republican National Committee recently improved upon this theory of divine authority to tyrannise, in these words : ' There is in this country a religious faith which believes in the divine origin of the constitution of the United States '.

" In our social organism most of us are acting like Christian Scientists. The fiction is that there is no pain, no social illness . . . The fact is that some parts of our social organism is suffering intensely."[1]

Religio-Therapeutic Type

Among the founders of new movements, we find an especially large number of persons who manifest various symptoms of the God-complex. These in fancy elevate themselves into the position of God ; in other words, they prefer themselves to the father and put themselves in the place usually reserved for an idealization of his image. This is observably true of P. P. Quimby, Mrs Eddy, and several writers on New Thought.

Quimby

In Quimby, for instance, one has not to read far before coming upon evidence that this innovator regarded himself as the embodiment of an all-seeing wisdom which was not vouchsafed to ordinary mortals. He claims :

" I found that ideas were matter condensed into a solid called disease, and that this solid like a book, contained all the wisdom of its author [i.e. it contained as much wisdom as the sick person might possess]. Seeing the book —for sight with wisdom embraces all the senses—I open it and see through it. To the patient it is a sealed book, but to wisdom there is nothing hid which cannot be revealed or seen."[2]

[1] Schroeder (Th.), " Emotional Conflicts, Liberty and Authority," *Psyche and Eros*, New York, January, 1923.
[2] *Quimby MSS.*, August, 1861. Quoted by Dresser (A. G.), *Phil. of P. P. Quimby*, p. 79.

Such wisdom (like salt) is connected in popular beliefs with the ideas of immortality (or eternity)[1] and incorruptibility, namely god-likeness, as also with the peculiarly divine or paternal quality of sexual potency.[2]

In the writings of Quimby we further find such tell-tale hints of his repressed attitude to his father as this :

> " When man . . . speaks a scientific truth, he is out of matter, and so far equal to God."[3]

At another time, he deifies the therapeutic system which is identified with himself :

> " This which I put in practice I call Christ acting through the man Quimby."[4]

Again, he avers that the essential person in each of us sons owes his birth to none but himself (the father not essential) :

> " The real man is God, as the first cause."[5]

Evidently the repressed meaning of these phrases did not escape Quimby's contemporaries, for he admits :

> " I am often accused of making myself equal with Christ."[6]

---

[1] " In connection with eternity is also mentioned the idea of wisdom, which salt likewise is supposed to symbolize. . . . ' Opinions both of divines and philosophers concur in making salt the *emblem of wisdom and learning*. . . . As it consists of the purest matter, so ought wisdom to be pure, sound, immaculate and incorruptible.' " Jones (E.), " The Symbolic Significance of Salt." In his *Essays in Applied Psycho-Analysis* (London, 1923), pp. 113-4.

[2] " The mere fact that salt has been regarded as the emblem of immortality and wisdom is in itself suggestive . . . for the other well-known emblem of these two concepts is the snake, which is in mythology and elsewhere the phallic symbol *par excellence*." Jones (E.), " The Symbolic Significance of Salt ", in his *Essays in Applied Psycho-Analysis* (London, 1923), p. 135.

[3] *Quimby MSS.*, 1861. Dresser (A. G.), *Phil. of P. P. Quimby*, p. 107.

[4] Quimby (P. P.), Dresser (H. W.), *Quimby MSS.*, p. 407.

[5] *Quimby MSS.*, 1865. Dresser (A. G.), *Phil. of P. P. Quimby*, p. 109.

[6] Quimby (P. P.), Dresser (H. W.), *Quimby MSS.*, p. 350.

Quimby's certainty that he possessed an *omnipotence of thought* available for the cure of his patients,[1] is hardly to be explained without assuming in him a modicum of the God-complex which is, in part, an identification with the parent to whom the infant attributes supreme and magical potency.   The healer in question, indeed, considered that he was able to cure only by becoming the father's mouthpiece, absorbing the father's words, and so speaking with his voice :

"Phineas Parkhurst Quimby . . . read much. The Bible was ever in his mind, and sometimes Berkeley."[2]

Mrs Eddy

Likewise must the Christian Scientist identify himself with the father (mind, God) in order to be magically potent for the exorcism of disease.   To depend on his mere human self, or to supplement the invocation of the father's spirit by materialistic therapy (thereby implying imperfect identification with him or trust in him) would be to break the spell.

"What seemed to be disease, vice and mortality are illusions of the physical senses . . . But the demonstration of the Science of Mind Healing by no means rests on the strength of human belief.   This demonstration is based on a true understanding of God . . .

" The lecturer, teacher, or healer who is indeed a Christian Scientist, never introduces the subject of human anatomy ; never depicts the muscular, vascular or nervous operations of the human frame.   He never talks about the structure of the human body.   He never lays his hands on the patient, nor manipulates the parts of the body supposed to be ailing."[3]

[1] " After reading your letter I tried to exercise all the power I was master of to quiet and restore your limb to health . . . I will . . . disturb your mind or fluids once more, and try to direct them to a more healthy state by repeating some of my ideas."   Quimby (P. P.), " Letter to Mrs Norcross ", in the *Quimby Manuscripts*, p. 81.

[2] Powell (Lyman), *Christian Science* (New York and London, 1917), p. 59.

[3] Eddy (Mrs M. A. M. B. G. P.), *Rudimentary Divine Science* (Boston, 1918), pp. 11-12,

The very existence of material things, so far as they imply that there is anything else in the universe than the father's spirit, must be categorically denied, according to the conception which Mrs Eddy received through Quimby from Berkeley:

" Question : What is the scientific statement of being ?

" Answer : No life, substance or intelligence in matter. That all is mind and there is no matter . . . Matter is unreal and mortal."[1]

In Mrs Eddy the God-complex is continuously evident. Her written word is to be read as a parallel volume, on a basis of equality with God's word. If anything, her word is to be the more authoritative of the two, since it defines the meaning of the other, and since no Christian Science reader may make any further comment of his own upon it as preachers in ordinary churches do upon the word merely of God.

Before her divinity, ordinary mortals stand eclipsed. She may at any time reduce the most exalted to the status of a domestic servant in her house, for (appropriating to herself the language of the Christ-father) " he that

[1] Eddy (Mrs M. A. M. B. G. P.), *Science of Man* (Boston, 1876), p. 8. To the same purpose is her assertion :—
" All is mind. According to the Scriptures and Christian Science all is God and there is nought beside Him. . . .
" The five material senses testify to the existence of matter. The spiritual senses afford no such evidence, but deny the testimony of the material senses. Which testimony is correct ? . . . If, as the Scriptures imply, God is All-in-All, then it must be Mind, since God is Mind. Therefore in Divine Science there is no material mortal man. . . .
" There is no material sense. . . . If there is any such thing as matter, it must be either mind which is called matter, or matter without mind.
" Matter without mind is a moral impossibility. . . . The body does not see, hear, smell, or taste. . . . Destroy this belief of seeing with the eye, and we could not see materially.
" Destroy the five senses as organized matter, and you must either become non-existent, or exist in mind only ; and this latter conclusion is the simple solution of the problem of being, and leads to the equal inference that there is no matter." Eddy (Mrs M. A. M. B. G. P.), *Rudimentary Divine Science* (Boston, 1918), p. 1.

loveth father or mother better than me is not worthy of me ".[1]

As Mrs Eddy seemed to set herself up as, if anything, superior to the authors of the Bible, so also Trine in one phrase gives Jesus rather a second place with himself :

> " In the dedicatory ' Message to My Readers ', Mr Trine assures us that the ' priceless possession ' he is trying to give us all is ' the inspiration and power ' involved in ' the Christianizing of the Christ '. "[2]

Mrs Eddy, who capitalized Quimby's system as the new religion of Christian Science, was not behind her instructor in the importance she attributed to herself and her books.   This characteristic appeared before ever she met Quimby ; her biographer relates how

> " She lived with one relative for a time, and then passed on to the next who would receive her.   Poor relation as she was in every home, she acted as though her presence was a privilege to be impressed on those with whom she lived. She took the best they had to give as though it were her right.   She had the family life adjusted to her nerves.   She made herself the ·centre of each situation.   She gave the servants extra trouble if there were servants in the house. If there were not, she let it sometimes fall upon a hostess old enough to be her mother.
> " If the thought of helping on as others do who fall into her plight, ever crossed her mind, she carefully safeguarded it from practical expression.   To spend your time writing books and entertaining callers while your hostess plays the drudge, to queen it at the sewing circle and ' lodge ' when there are duties to be done at the home where you are staying, does not tend to the perpetuation of the welcome . . . So in all those bitter years, which ran on from 1843 to 1870,

---

[1] " If the author of the Christian Science text-book calls on this Board for household help or a handmaid, the Board shall immediately appoint a proper member of this Church therefor, and the appointee shall go immediately in obedience to the call.
  " ' He that loveth father or mother more than me is not worthy of me '. "   Eddy (Mrs M. A. M. B. G. P.), *Church Manual* (Boston, 1924), p. 69.
[2] Bedborough (Geo.), *Harmony or Humbug : an Examination of Mr Ralph Waldo Trine's Book, In Tune with the Infinite* (Letchworth, 1917).

Mrs Eddy was engaged almost continuously in wearing out her welcome."[1]

Her books, she says, will bless humanity[2] and revolutionize the world[3], and are too sacred to be commented on by ordinary mortals.[4]

New Thought Writers

The God-complex is also shared by many founders of the New Thought branch of Quimbian metaphysics. R. W. Trine seems to speak out of familiarity with it :

" And what is a God-man ? One in whom the powers of God are manifesting, through a man. No one can set limitations to a man or woman of this type ; for the only limitations he or she can have are those set by the self."[5]

The implication that he has himself experienced identification with the father is still more explicit when Trine volunteers to tell us how easy it is for everyone of us to accomplish that feat :

[1] Powell (Lyman), *Christian Science* (New York and London, 1917), pp. 56-7.

[2] " Reading my books without prejudice would convince all that their purpose is right. The comprehension of my teachings would enable anyone to prove these books to be filled with blessings for the whole human family." Eddy (Mrs M. A. M. B. G. P.), *No and Yes* (Boston, 1918), p. 15.

[3] " If the Bible and my work, *Science and Health*, had their rightful place in schools of learning, they would revolutionize the world." Eddy (Mrs M. A. M. B. G. P.), *No and Yes* (Boston, 1918), p. 33.

[4] " SECT IV. The first readers in the Christian Science Churches shall read the correlative texts in *Science and Health with Key to the Scriptures* ; and the second readers shall read the Bible texts. . . .
" SECT V. The readers of *Science and Health with Key to the Scriptures*, before commencing to read from this book, shall distinctly announce the full title of the book and give the author's name. . . .
" SECT VI. These readers . . . shall make no remarks explanatory of the Lesson Sermon at any time, but they shall read all notices and remarks that may be printed in the *Christian Science Quarterly.*" Eddy (Mrs M. A. M. B. G. P.), *Church Manual of the First Church of Christ Scientist* (Boston, 1924), p. 32.
" No member shall use written formulas nor permit his patients or pupils to use them, as auxiliaries to teaching Christian Science or for healing the sick. Whatever is requisite for either is contained in the books of the Discoverer and Founder of Christian Science." Eddy (Mrs M. A. M. B. G. P.), *Church Manual* (Boston, 1924), p. 43.

[5] Trine (R. W.), *In Tune with the Infinite* (London, 1923), p. 8.

"In the degree that we open ourselves to this divine inflow we are changed from mere men into God-men."[1]

"In the degree that we open ourselves to this divine inflow, does . . . this voice of intuition . . . this voice of God speak clearly . . . until by-and-by there comes the time when it is unerring, absolutely unerring."[2]

The same writer also manifests his God-complex when he says :

"We never could have been, and never can be, other than Divine Being. And I fully agree with . . . Max Müller . . . 'Man cannot, say, become God, because he is God. What else could he be, if God is the only true and real being ? ' "[3]

Another interesting thing about this quotation is the title of the book in which it appears. For it suggests childhood's queries about the subject of birth, a subject which adults keep so secret that it might well be called by this same title, *The Greatest Thing Ever Known* ".[4]

Another New Thought writer, Orison Swett Marden, has entitled one of his books, *Every Man a King*—i.e. in the language of the unconscious, everyone the equal of the father. In another of his works we learn that :

" The sons and daughters of God were planned for glorious, sublime lives, and the time will come when all men will be kings, and all women queens . . . The plan of creation will have failed if every human being does not finally come into his own and return to his God as king." (Read, return to his father as himself one of the fathers).[5]

Of a piece with the talk we have often heard from Quimby and Mrs Eddy about *error*, and with the whole

---

[1] *Idem*, p. 9.

[2] *Idem*, p. 28.

[3] Such is the magnitude of the potency which Trine is able to realize through self-identification with God, that :—

"Even animals feel the effect of these forces. . . . Therefore, whenever we meet an animal, we can do it good by sending out to it these thoughts of love. It will feel the effects whether we simply entertain them or whether we voice them." Trine (R. W.), *In Tune with the Infinite* (London, 1923), pp. 72-3.

[4] Trine (R. W.), *Greatest Thing Ever Known* (London, 1898), p. 10.

[5] Marden (O. S.), *Peace, Power and Plenty* (London, 1923).

I

attitude of denial of the tangible and of every basis of real science (so that the world is reduced to a nursery room in which baby imagines that if he were his potent father, he could destroy or create anything imaginable by mere wishing)—of a piece with all this is Trine's assertion that no reality exists outside of opinion :

> " The optimist is right. The pessimist is right. The one differs from the other as the light from the dark. Yet both are right . . . Point of view is the determining factor in the life of each. It determines as to whether it is a life of power or of *impotence.*"[1]

Orison Swett Marden is another who feels that, as father's boy, it must be that he shares some of father's immunity to the petty accidents that plague other and naughtier children. It should be noted that dreams about fire are in childhood the regular accompaniment of bed-wetting,[2] and this would indeed be an accident from which the father is immune. Marden asks :

> " What have panics, or fires, or financial losses to do with the well-balanced man whom God made ? . . . I do not believe that the coming man, the man of the highest civiliza-tion would be any more affected by the entire destruction of all his property than the laws of harmony would be affected by the burning up of all the musical instruments in the world."[3]

This paragraph is taken from the book, *Every Man a King* (or father). It is followed on the next page by a (to the psychologist) delightful flight of fancy, in which Marden prophecies that some day people will become wealthy, not by working and saving, but by repressing the reality-sense and (to use a vulgarism) " kidding " themselves along. This is perhaps essentially a mastur-bation-phantasy of self-sufficiency toward pleasure, an

---

[1] Trine (R. W.), *In Tune with the Infinite* (London, 1923), p. 1. (Italics mine).

[2] Probably the association is through the burning sensation of the excretions on the skin, and also through the opposition of the ideas of fire and water.

[3] Marden (O. S.), *Every Man a King* (London), pp. 236-7.

Aladdin's lamp dream, but may well also receive energy from the child's thought that, if he were the father, he would be (in comparison with other children) very rich indeed[1] and that, by no process which the child clearly understands. Here is Marden's prophecy :

" The coming man will always be prosperous because he will not allow the poverty thought, the limitation thought, to enter his mind. He will always hold thoughts of prosperity and abundance."[2]

Adherents of these schools are very emphatic upon the power for evil or good which is exerted by depressed or cheerful thinking. Thus, Trine :

" The pessimist, by virtue of his own limitations, is making his own hell, and . . . helping to make one for all mankind."[3]

That optimist-at-any-price, Marden, predicts :

" The coming man will not have the word ' can't ' in his vocabulary, for he will not have any doubts in his mind."[4]

In Couéism we find the same optimistic sense of potency expressed with only a shade less extravagance :

" Be sure that you will obtain what you want, and you will obtain it, so long as it is within reason."[5]

There is, to be sure, rather more of an attempt to put these hopes upon the basis of some scientific explanation, by attributing them to the consequences which our thinking has upon our own personal efficiency,[6] and less

---

[1] The reader will recall the quatrain in R. L. Stevenson's *Child's Garden of Verses* :
> " When I am grown to man's estate
> I shall be very proud and great
> And tell the other girls and boys
> Not to meddle with my toys."

[2] Marden (O. S.), *Every Man a King*, p. 238.
[3] Trine (R. W.), *In Tune with the Infinite* (London, 1923), p. 1.
[4] Marden (O. S.), *Every Man a King*, p. 238.
[5] Leon (Mme Emile), *Thoughts and Precepts of Emile Coué* (London, 1922), p. 38.
[6] " Every thought entirely filling our mind becomes true for us and tends to transform itself into action." Coué (E.), *Self Mastery* (London, 1922), p. 19.

to mystical harmonies assumed to exist between ourselves and the outside universe. But in their emphasis on the importance of auto suggestion, all of these schools are emphasising the value (as they consider) of continual reference to that *super-ego* which was shown by Freud to be in the first instance generated through attempts at identification with the father.[1]

The motive of omnipotence of thought is so obviously present in Coué — as in the Christian Science and New Thought camps—that a single illustration will suffice.

Without any qualification, Coué reduces the problems of medicine and sociology to the single factor of opinion, in this sentence :

" If you can make a sick person think that her trouble is getting better, it will disappear ; if you succeed in making a kleptomaniac think that he will cease to steal," etc., etc.[2]

So much for the suggestive therapeuts and their sense of omnipotence. But I will mention another instance of the God-complex.

A cult which, with its curious mixture of modern and ancient ideas, of common sense and of pseudo-oriental terminology, is gaining a fair number of adherents in America and Europe, is Mazdaznan.

Otto Hanish, who quitted the humble calling of butcher's errand boy to develop into the prophet of the Mazdaznan cult, has rechristened himself Ottoman Zar

---

[1] We shall refer under the next caption to Jones' demonstration of how auto-suggestion is thus ultimately, like ordinary suggestion, operative through the attachment to the father.

[2] Coué (E.), *Self Mastery* (London, 1922), p. 19.
A more nearly sane statement is this one : " Whoever starts in life with the idea ' I shall succeed ', always succeeds, because he does what is necessary to bring about this result." Leon (Mme E.), *Thoughts and Precepts of Emile Coué* (London, 1922), p. 39.
More questionably, " to become master of oneself it is enough to think that one is becoming so ".

Adusht H'nish. In one of his books he even signs himself royally

> " With the blessing of all good things,
>> " OTTOMAN,
>>> " Prince of Adusht."[1]

It may be objected by some persons, that to have shown that Otto Hanish or any others of the leaders of the movements we are discussing owed their beliefs to certain complexes, does not prove that any large portion of the mass of their followers to-day are not impelled to these beliefs purely from rational motives. Against such a position, I can only urge the saneness of Ernest Jones' contention :

> " A person brought up in however superstitious a society would not develop a given superstition unless it was of such a kind as to be capable of being associated to his personal mental complexes. This association is a purely individual one, and without it the superstitious belief fails to appeal ; it need hardly be said that the process, particularly in civilized communities, is most often entirely unconscious."[2]

The belief that one has succeeded, or will succeed, to the place of the father—whose power seems truly magical to the child—is fertile ground for the belief in the omnipotence of one's own thoughts. And such a belief plainly plans an immense rôle in Christian Science, New Thought, and Couéism.

As we have seen in this chapter, then, a doubleness of attitude has prevailed co-operatives and communists, and on the part of Marx, Lenin, socialists and the democrats. The sense of omnipotence, if not actually the God-complex, was plainly a moving force in Quimby, Mrs Eddy, Trine, Marden and Coué.

---

[1] Hanish (O. Z.), *Mazdaznan Health and Breath Culture*, p. 185.
[2] Jones (E.), *The Symbolic Significance of Salt*, published in *Imago*, 1912, Bd. I, S. 361 and 454 ; republished in hi : *Essays in Applied Psycho-Analysis* (London, 1923), p. 202.

PART II

PRO-FATHER MOTIVES

PART II

CHAPTER I

ANXIETY, CONSCIENCE, SENSE OF SIN, SELF-ABASEMENT AND SELF-PUNISHMENT

INTRODUCTORY REMARKS

THE present chapter begins that part of this thesis which will deal with motives that prompt us to act congruently with the father's wishes, and to oppose those who rebel against him. But such motives are not necessarily at bottom derived from genuine love of the father. They may be only reaction-formations against repressed hate of him.

Hatred openly recognized may be dealt with in a rational manner, as where Shakespeare's Prospero declaims :

> " With my nobler reason 'gainst my fury
> Do I take part. The rarer action is
> In virtue than in vengeance."[1]

It is not, however, with such cases that we are called upon to deal here, but with instances where the underlying hatred is inhibited from being cognized by the primary consciousness. For then it either assumes disguised forms to evade the censor, or else the repressing forces, remaining solely in evidence, excuse their presence where no true opponent is seen to exist, by attaching themselves to a fictitious objective.

A child is punished when he expresses his anti-social

[1] Shakespeare, *The Tempest*, V. i. 27.

feelings. Usually the task of inflicting this punishment
falls upon the father. Threats also are made to the
child that unless he is good, father will chastise him.
Excessive zeal in such means of correction may cause
irrational fears, as well as have its part in the genesis of
conscience and also of the sense of sin.

Genesis of Irrational Fears

Since the real father cannot be everywhere and see
everything, fictitious fathers are invented who may be
supposed to possess these powers : Father Christmas,
the Bogey Man, the Devil, God, etc. Then the knowledge that he has been guilty of wicked thoughts may
serve to call up images of these father surrogates, and,
with them, the anxiety or fear which the boy used to feel
when his real father stood by to punish.[1]

Gould (whom I have frequently named in these
pages), describing a dream accompanied by a strong
sense of fear, said, " After awakening, a picture of a
former physical combat with my brother presented
itself ". The brother, however, was only a lay figure,
and the combat with him screened a more serious
estrangement from his father.

Fears arising in this way are out of all proportion to
the fictitious object upon which they are projected, and
precisely because their real and adequate object remains

[1] Pfister relates how :
" A schoolmistress brought me a little boy, seven years old.
" He suffered from sleeplessness and distressing dreams. . . . When
he awoke at night it seemed to him as if someone were coming . . . a
man dressed in black, with a long white beard and pale face. Burning
eyes. Angry. . . . Yes, Father Christmas. . . . He catches naughty
little boys.
" In his sleepless hours he often thinks of how he does not love his
mother, because she is always scolding and punishing him. He wants
to pay her out. . . . If his mother has been angry with him, he can
punish her by being naughty at school. . . . If he has bad reports
this will vex his mother.
" Thus the anxiety arises partly from an uneasy conscience, but
partly from the need of atonement. Father Christmas will punish
him severely for his wrong doing." Pfister (O.), *Love in Children*
(London, 1924), p. 280.

hidden. Dangers are even invented, or are regarded as real and present when, as a matter of fact, they are remote or even speculative.

From the question of anxieties and fears let us pass to the closely related one of conscience. For, as we have already noted, this is a reverberation of the father's commands as they were authoritatively impressed upon our receptive infant mind :

> " In the orthodox Christian conception, the good life is the virtuous life, and virtue consists in obedience to the will of God, and the will of God is revealed to each individual through the voice of conscience. This whole conception is that of men subject to an alien despotism."[1]

Phineas Quimby—whom we have already found to have been gifted with flashes of insight—observed of his patients' illnesses that

> " Some cases have been occasioned by the idea that they had committed the unpardonable sin. When asked what it was, no two persons answered alike."[2]

But Quimby failed to draw from this fact the conclusions which would have placed him a half century in advance of his time. For we find him only repeating the old theological explanation :

> " The sick are merely slaves of superstition, made so by the sins of their parents."[3]

This sense of illness and impotence (castration) being the fitting punishment for having harboured wishes against the father is repeated in *Christian Science* :

> " If you are fettered by sin you are unfit to free another from the fetters of disease."[4]

[1] Russell (B.), " Salvation ; Individual and Social," in *What I Believe* (London, 1925); pp. 67-8.
[2] *Quimby MSS.*, September, 1861. Dresser (A. G.), *Philosophy of P. P. Quimby*, p. 81.
[3] *Quimby MSS.*, Dresser (H. W.), *The Quimby MSS.*, p. 296.
[4] Eddy (Mrs M. A. M. B. G. P.), *Science and Health With Key to the Scriptures* (Jerusalem, 1924), p. 194.

The idea appears also frequently in the literature of New Thought. The fear of *talion* from the revengeful father (it was he who was the earliest avenger in the experience of most of us) is evident in slightlysublimated form in the following passage from Ralph Waldo Trine :

> " If the thought forces sent out by any particular life are those of hatred or jealousy or malice or fault-finding or criticism or scorn, these same thought forces are aroused and sent back from others so that one is affected not only by reason of the unpleasantness of having such thoughts from others, but they also in turn affect one's own mental states, and through these his own bodily conditions, so that as far as the welfare of self is concerned, the indulgences in thoughts and emotions of this nature are most expensive, most detrimental, most destructive."[1]

> " You never can tell what your thoughts will do
>   In bringing you hate or love,
> And they speed on the track to bring you back
>   Whatever went out from your mind."[2]

Although more sublimated, the same motive, it appears to me, is still at work in Trine's recognition and formulation of what, doubtless, comes near to being a fact :

> " There is no such thing as finding true happiness by searching for it directly . . . So there is no such thing as finding true greatness by searching for it directly."[3]

Self-punishment-wishes seem also the only explanation of this remark by another leader of the movement, Horatio Dresser :

> " True, if one could conquer every woe, one would be decidedly a loser. No one wants to be a Stoic."[4]

Spiritism is the surviving form of the once widespread belief that dead ancestors return to punish the living for the evil wishes harboured against them. In some

[1] Trine (R. W.), *What all the World's A-Seeking* (London, 1900), p. 29.
[2] *Idem*, p. 32.
[3] *Idem*, p. 13.
[4] Dresser (H. W.), *Book of Secrets* (New York, 1902), pp. 53-4.

cases the tables are turned, and it is the parent who, having sent his boy away to be killed in the war, is now haunted by the latter's spirit. This, and not only the wish to see again those we loved, may help to explain many war-time ghosts and other supernatural phenomena. The movement had a tremendous popularity during the latter half of the 19th century, and almost as great a revival immediately after the war, when the deaths of so many fathers and sons must have aroused powerful complexes in those who loved but yet at the same time secretly hated them. Some fathers loudly bragged of having sent their sons to the battlefield.

Conscience

Returning to the subject of conscience, the following is a definition of it in fairly orthodox terms :

" Conscience is nothing else than the echo of God's voice within the soul."

This is psychologically correct, in view of the equation God = father. Conscience may interfere pathologically in a sphere in which it is wholly out of place, namely in estimating the truth or falsity of some hypothesis. In a criticism of psycho-analysis, which I am about to cite from an encyclopædia, the motive of the writer, a Roman Catholic, appears to be revealed in the first line. He believes that the repression of wicked inclinations is *demanded by the moral law*, i.e. by the voice of the heavenly father. From that point onward, he becomes not the impartial investigator of reality (to which indeed he makes no reference during the whole argument) but an advocate concerned only to deny any facts which contradict the voice of his father. A conflict in his own psyche between a rebellious sense of reality and the dominant Conscience, is indicated by the extraordinary series of imaginary facts which he proceeds to conjure up, all *a priori*, and without offering evidence for any of them. Besides misstatements of his opponents' position, there is " sprung " on us, in practically every sentence, a hitherto undiscovered law of psychology :

> " The conscious repression demanded by the moral law will prevent the formation of hidden complexes and will exercise deliberate control over evil impulses and tendencies. Habits of virtue, moreover, will not only repress the wicked inclinations into the unconscious, but will drain them of all their energy and gradually supplant them entirely. The most important fact overlooked by psycho-analysts is this, that disorders of the mental life are not so much caused by effectually repressed desires as by insufficiently suppressed desires which are allowed to lurk in the mind. The Christian law forbidding evil thoughts prevents such insincerity that may avenge itself in psychic disturbances.
>
> " Psycho-analysis contains elements of truth, but they are distorted beyond recognition by the fantastic and pseudo-scientific terminology affected by the apostles of the new theory. Many of its heralded discoveries are common sense truths expressed in a mysterious jargon calculated to impress the uneducated . . . Catholic asceticism has long anticipated what is useful in psycho-analysis, which has not even clarified the matters in question . . .
>
> " . . . The unconscious is neither dynamic nor as omnipresent as the psycho-analyst would make it out. Freud has entirely inverted psychology, making the unconscious the dominant factor in our psychic life and exalting the instinctive life above the rational . . . On this point, psycho-analysis is in accord with the general drift of modern evolutionary psychology."[1]

" Thus " we are tempted to quote in view of this writer's retreat into a refuge of absurd statements, " conscience doth make cowards of us all ". We refuse to face going counter to our awe of the father.

Not only do we continue in after years to hear the echo of the father's voice commanding this or forbidding that ; not only is our conduct still modelled after patterns which were stamped in by punishments during infancy, but we adopt his voice as our own, and we hold up the pattern thus formed as our ideal. This

[1] Bruche (C.), art. " Psycho-Analysis ", in *Catholic Encyclopædia Supplement*, I.

process commences in the little boy when he sets up his father as a model to copy.

Conscience is, then, the voice of the father speaking through the medium of the super-ego.[1] That his voice may become harsh to the verge of unreasonableness follows as a corollary. It will go to an extreme of exaction at which the father himself would have stopped short. For instance, it makes us feel it is more sinful to harbour lustful thoughts against the mother, or to take the name of God (father) in vain, than it would be to commit some act really disastrous to the well-being of the community.

The father representing, even more than the mother, in most families, the principle of authority, and the denial of the pleasure principle, restraint was felt in his presence and became associated with him. In after life the presence of temptation calls up the father's prohibition and this restraint feeling which accompanied past experiences.

The saying, " the voice of conscience is the voice of God ", very clearly portrays a sense of the paternal origin of conscience. Conscience comes in to call a halt when there arise desires to disobey authoritative (paternal) moral rules.[2]

These things, like power, and the distinction of being a possessor, the son secretly would like to snatch from

[1] " From the later stages of development of the ego . . . a special faculty is slowly formed . . . able to oppose the rest of the ego, with the function of observing and criticising the self and exercising a censorship within the mind, and this we become aware of as our ' conscience '. Freud (S.) : *Collected Papers*, vol. IV, p. 388.

" It would not surprise us if we were to find a special institution in the mind which performs the task of seeing that narcissistic gratification is secured from the ego-ideal and . . . watches the real ego and measures it by that ideal. . . . That which we call our *conscience* has the required characteristics. . . .

" That which prompted the person to form an ego-ideal, over which his conscience keeps guard, was the influence of parental criticism." *Idem.*, pp. 52-53.

" Conscience and morality arose through over-coming, de-sexualizing, the Œdipus-complex " *Idems*, vol. II, p. 266.

[2] Freud (S.), " The Economic Problem in Masochism ". First pub. in *Zeitschrift*, Bd. X, 1924. Transl. Riviere. Repub. in *Collected Papers*, vol. II, (London, 1925).

the father. Against such tendencies he is likely to over-compensate with a superstitious dread, the intensity of which corresponds to that of his desires. Disaster will surely overtake him if he touches these things.

The wish to be self-born, or at least born without owing anything to our father, disguises itself sometimes in a most clever way in a desire to be regenerated. Thus by an assumption that the purpose of our wish is to be more as our father would have been ambitious to see us, we manage to smuggle past the censor a desire originally directed against him.

Sin

Where the person has gone counter to the dictates of his conscience, or, in other words, to the inner echo of his father's voice, he experiences a sense of guilt and sin. Sin is essentially a feeling of conflict between father-regarding, and rebellious, desires.

Freud has told us how the sense of *original sin* arises from a reaction against the Œdipus complex. It apparently is a frequent factor in the way in which criminals who take extreme precautions to cover up all traces of their crime, will yet thwart themselves by leaving one perfectly obvious clue uncovered, so that capture is certain. This same self-contradictory un-witting desire to be punished for one's guilty wishes against the father may well be a contributory factor in the readiness of the young to " prove themselves " in the initiations devised by their elders, both in primitive and in advanced communities.

The accusations of the conscience-stricken son against his own lack of filial piety often takes the form of self-vilification.[1] " I am a poor, miserable sinner," etc. Now, humanity is an extension of self. In some ways it therefore better suits our self esteem to displace our revilings from self on to the enlarged self, humanity. Instead of saying " I am incorrigible ", we say, " you can't change human nature ".

[1] Therefore the rebel Ruskin says : " First be sure your conscience is not an ass."

If the father dies, this event, because it is so in accord with some of the son's wishes, gives the son a sense of having partly caused that death. (Omnipotence of thought.) So he imagines that the spirit of the dead comes back to haunt him. Among savages this is a foundation of spiritism. Cursed with this indefinable sense of " original sin ", " the unforgivable sin ", etc., one feels he must atone to God (father).

The immediate effect of a sense of sin will generally be a strong over-compensation in the direction of a professed repudiation of all rebellious tendencies, going so far as to deny that we have any rights or dignity at all. Thus we get self-abasement.

Less recognised than the above is the fact, that conscience is continually compelling us to conduct, the chief or only purpose of which is self-punishment. The child has been taught to feel that when it has done wrong it must suffer chastisement. In adult-hood there often is no outside person to administer such punishment. But to make the situation *as if* childhood were here again—the adult is incessantly desiring this—the repressed nature of the man arranges that some disaster shall befall through maladroit behaviour.

> " Conscious guilt is intense in proportion to the discrepancy between the wishes of the real ego and the standards of the ego-ideal.
> " But to an unsuspected extent the operations of this conscience system are carried on beneath the level of the conscious personality . . . and here, strangest of all, it brings about what we call unconscious self-punishment."[1]

[1] Further : "Conscious conscience . . . observes, criticises, and at times compels the ego to do penance for breaches of adult standards, and in this respect is infinitely more concerned over *actual* breaches of such standards. . . . The unconscious conscience on the other hand, does not distinguish to the same extent between deed and intention. It began to operate when the child, like primitive man, believed in the magical efficacy of thought and wish. Certain neurotic sufferers are burdened with an intolerable sense of guilt and tendencies to self reproach, which they cannot adequately explain on conscious grounds, which they are compelled to explain in terms of the most trivial actual occurrences. , , . When such cases are investigated psycho-analytic-

Freud remarks that the self accusations of the pious correspond notably to those of the obsessional neurotic. It is well known that such a sense of sin has led whole populations to outbreaks of self-punitive orgies (such as those of the flagellants during the middle ages) and to the advocacy of such extreme doctrines of obedience and self-abasing submissiveness as were held by the Jesuits. The latter taught (but it should be noted that the homage to Father God is not so real as that to Mother Church) :

" We should submit ourselves to the church so completely that if we clearly perceived a thing to be white and she were to declare it black, we should, with her, declare it black."[1]

ally, it is found that they are restraining and punishing themselves for imaginary crimes existing only in the form of unconscious wishes." Glover (James), "Man, The Individual", in *Social Aspects of Psy. An.* (London, 1924), ed. by E. Jones, pp. 65-6.
" The protestations of the pious that they know that they are miserable sinners in their hearts, corresponds to the sense of guilt of the obsessional neurotic ; while the pious observances (prayers, invocations, etc.) with which they begin every act of the day, and especially every unusual undertaking, seem to have the significance of defensive and protective measures." Freud (S.), " Obsessive Acts and Practices." First pub. in the *Zeitschrift für Religionspsychologie*, Bd. I, 1907. Reprinted in *Collected Papers* (London, 1924), vol. II, p. 31.
[1] " Spiritual Exercises," quoted in *Maxims of St Ignatius Loyala*, p. 99.
A friend whose relationships with his extremely religious father were characterized by excessive submission and obedience, varied with acts which revealed repressed rebelliousness, and who subsequently developed neurotic tendencies, has lent me an autobiographical manuscript. In this I find :—
" During a holiday at Millport, when I was about ten, I remember walking by the seashore and listening to the long roll of the surf. It seemed to me that a voice within me said, ' I curse the Holy Ghost '. Then in a flash came the terrible thought. I had committed the unforgivable sin ! This preyed on my mind for many months ; till one evening my father found me crying in bed and asked the reason. I told him I was lost and had committed the unforgivable sin. . . .
" It is strange to me that I was only really happy when I forgot religion. While birdnesting, playing truant, and penetrating the mysterious recesses of the quarries near our home, I was carefree and undisturbed by some strange power that seemed to force me in a certain direction against my will. Various nervous symptoms appeared at this time. There was a constant cough, difficulty in swallowing, acute dread of sitting in church, and heart palpitation. Church bells sent a sinking feeling all through me, and I longed to run away from everything associated with those nerve racking services." Peat (D. A.), *Shedding the Husk*. An autobiographical manuscript, lent to the present writer in November, 1925.

Economico-Political Type of Movements

An attitude of self-subordination so extreme as to arouse the certainty that it is a reaction formation against rebellious wishes almost equally strong, appears in many monkish writings, and, too, in a quarter whence we should little expect it to emanate—namely socialist sources.

Thus R. Blatchford declares, with a piety which calls up pictures of rosaries and sandalled feet :

> " Just as no man can have a right to the land, because no man makes the land, so no man has a right to his self, because he did not make that self."[1]

A similar sense of the unworthiness of us miserable sinners and of the need of grace to be had through renunciation, inspires a sentence in Fabian Tract No. 127 :

> " No one should or could have the right to ask that he shall be employed at the particular job which suits his particular taste and temperament."[2]

In the introductory remarks to this chapter, we have already considered how the sense of the weakness of one's own character may be displaced on to poor human nature in general. The " you can't change human nature " argument is a tried and trusty one against all social innovations, it having been used even to check the introduction of popular elementary education. A somewhat changed form of this displaced humility is given below. The identification of civilization with the father, which will be found in it, is probably due to its author conceiving civilization in the abstract as meaning capitalism. (The man, whose name I shall conceal, calling him " X——", was very conservative.)

> " The fact that civilization has not produced complete happiness, satisfaction, or complete justice for all men and women, is due, not to civilization, but to human nature."[3]

---

[1] Blatchford (R.), *Merrie England*, ed. 1908, p. 87, quoted in *Anti-Socialist Speakers' Handbook*, p. 18.
[2] *Socialism and the Labour Party*. Fabian Tract, no. 127, p. 7. Quoted in *Anti-Socialist Speakers' Handbook*.
[3] " X——", *F. of a L.* (New York, 1924), p. 198,

How often all of us have heard the theological form of this argument : Evil is not God's fault but Man's : Evidently Civilization=Father—God.

The reader will recall that I have referred to an analysand by the name of Kenyon. In many respects I found his to be an enlightening instance—although of course only an individual one—of how attitudes may be determined by the negative aspects of the father-transference. Kenyon had scruples against using the money left him by his father, and against endorsing any rebel programme or movement wholeheartedly and without reservations.[1]

[1] Some years before the father's death, this forthcoming event became a favourite subject of speculation with the son. The latter, owing to his neurosis, had been unable to concentrate his energies upon any pursuit long enough to make a success of it. He suffered from a strong inferiority complex which defended him from the rebuff of feeling " I have tried my utmost and failed to show a grown man's capacity ", by always securing his withdrawal from any venture before he had really put forth his strength.

He had recently embarked on a business which, owing to his own shortcomings, was rapidly using up his available capital and the sums which his mother generously but unwisely advanced him. The prospective death of his father, which ultimately did bring him a large fortune in time to save the situation, came to be more and more cynically hoped for as the only escape from disaster and the entailed confession of incompetence.

Corresponding to this wish, however, there existed a powerful guilt complex. Desire for the death of the father for the sake of inheriting his fortune must somehow be justified to conscience. In this situation, the subject's sociological interests come to the rescue by suggesting the following rationalization :—

So long as the fortune remained in his father's hands it was being used towards no socially beneficial purpose beyond its own multiplication. Every additional year that the father survived, increased the chance that he might outlive the son, and therefore the money never would do any good in the world. If, however, the subject himself were to become possessed of the estate, he would apply it to altruistic purposes. Consequently, the good of society demanded the immediate death of the father.

Now, in much revolutionary propaganda, we find a similar optimism and glorification of results expected to follow from success of some movements, e.g. it is claimed for proletarian or communist culture.

" Prolet-cult is the lamp whereby all the roads of advance are lighted." Paul (Eden and Cedar), *Prolet-Cult* (London), p. 18.

When actually Kenyon's father died, this was only a long anticipated event. As regularly happens under like circumstances, the son received the news without sorrow. More, he felt no subsequent remorse at his own death wishes, probably because they had been so openly acknowledged to himself,

RELIGIO-THERAPEUTIC TYPE OF MOVEMENTS

We might admit that certain insights into our own nature—insights of a slightly higher order than the mere recognition of immediate desires—may be hieroglyphed in the religious forms. But even if we were further to admit the worth ascribed by Silberer and others to *anagogic* interpretations of such material, yet the readiness to accept it as literally and objectively true is to-day unusual. Even as a code of morality the ancient body of lore has to be regarded as so inadequate to the com-

That a guilt complex nevertheless existed is witnessed to by the fact, that after the passage of twelve years, the son still refrains from touching for his own personal use, more than a minor part of the income of his father's estate.

The son's constructive interests ran a various gamut which finally transferred them from the mechanical into the social field. His interest in sociology alarmed the father, who accused him of leaning towards socialism. The son's knowledge of what socialism might be, was small ; but during the whole of his father's lifetime he remained under the influence of his father's contemptuous attitude toward the forbidden movement. Few experiences more violently irritated him than to be told, as he occasionally was by advocates of socialism, that he would eventually adopt that doctrine. Actually their prophecies proved to be not far wrong ; he is generally regarded as a socialist by others, though he still never calls himself so.

In fact, two years before his father's death, when life in a large city brought him into contact with these modern movements from all understanding of which school and college had hitherto screened him, he veered towards the most opposite extreme from socialism, by flirting with anarchism—a movement to which his father would have been still more hostile, but which he never had actually mentioned.

After his father's death, Kenyon swung so far away from the parental attitude on political and economic questions as to leave little doubt but that submission rather than love had held him hitherto. Indeed he had long been fully conscious of much terror lest his father should punish heterodoxy by cutting off his inheritance (perhaps an anal form of castration complex). He now began to interest himself in various movements of a revolutionary nature. He consorted with socialists, anarchists, syndicalists, and to a slight extent with communists. Yet echoes of parental disapproval still made it impossible to identify himself with any one group. He merely remained sympathetic with them all.

When he became engaged to be married, he stipulated with his fiancée that a compromise should be continued whereby both lived on not more than half of their income, and they have adhered to the agreement. The balance of the income has been given to various left wing movements. (The father arranged that the capital should remain in trust).

plexities of modern industrial and democratic society[1]
that defence of the old beliefs no longer often dares assert
such absurdities as we find in Comstock, in New Thought
Writers (with especially their efforts to exculpate the
father from responsibilities for evils) and some sthenic
doctrines.

Comstock

We therefore suspect motives not related to the reality-
principle in Anthony Comstock, who calls the beliefs of
our fathers :

" the fastenings which are the only restraints of vice."

This man, whose censoring proclivities have already
shown him to us as anti-son and pro-father, attacks as
follows a noted agnostic of his time :

> " Mr Ingersoll is much like the white elephant in a
> menagerie, in a story told by Rev C. H. Spurgeon, that
> broke loose and then opened the cages containing the lions
> and tigers . . . But Mr Ingersoll goes further. He not only
> breaks the fastenings which are the only restraints of vice,
> but by ridicule and laughter seeks to lull the watchman,
> Conscience, to sleep, so that the soul shall have no monitor
> to sound a warning.[2]

In all this there is a decided note of anxiety. The
thought that anyone could wish to banish the heavenly
father appears to have startled Comstock with such
alarm as a guilty conscience feels. In another passage

---

[1] " The future progress of human culture will demand a very considerable modification and purification of most existing religious forms.
The study of the psychology of religion is showing that these forms are,
for the most part, based on crude unconscious motives which have
to be outgrown and superseded if civilisation is to prosper and advance.
In retaining and fostering these forms we are in many cases playing
into hands, not of the higher, but of the baser and more primitive aspects
of our nature, aspects which, at our present level of development, it is
necessary indeed to understand, but not to venerate or even to approve." Flügel (J. C.), *The Psycho-Analytic Study of the Family*
(London, 1923).

[2] Comstock (A.), *Traps for the Young* (New York, 1884), pp. 185-6.

he likewise takes the position that father-rejection is, and must be, the cause of all debauchery. Unbelief is evidently greatly to be feared :

" In Wall Street I found a boy about twenty years of age, who had twenty varieties of the most debauching matter in his pockets. . . . His father . . . told me that his son was the only one of seven children who was not converted to God."[1]

The fear of unbelief readily passes over to fear of the process which most obviously conduces to that state, namely to fear of reason. Against the trustful obedient son is contrasted the argumentative son. It was when the son began to doubt and dispute with his father, that troubles began.

Thought-Cure

Some such memories must have influenced Quimby to make an assertion, the logical corollary of which would be, that spells of reflection would be followed by illness, and that public epidemics followed on periods of intellectual renaissance ! The assertion I refer to goes :

" Man, in his natural state, was no more liable to disease than the beast, but as soon as he began to reason he became diseased ; for his disease was in his reason."[2]

Coué also, apparently, has in some degree felt this inhibition against intellectuality. We are told that he did, indeed, have a bent towards chemistry, but that he presently

" turned toward that branch of science that calls for no apparatus or extra expense, namely, psychology. (Sic !)
" M Coué has always despised theory pure and simple . . . He has always been a man of action . . . The theory of psychology has never been his strong point."[3]

[1] *Idem*, pp. 140-1.
[2] Quimby,(P. P.), as quoted by Dresser (A. G.), *Philosophy of P. P. Quimby* (Boston, 1895), p. 65.
[3] Noble (Lady), *M. Coué and Auto-Suggestion* (Chatham and London, 1924), pp. 1-2.

So frequent, indeed, is the connection between religion and morbid fears, that upon the one hand the religious apologists regularly give as an argument *ad hominem* for their beliefs that these are a consolation against fears, while, on the other hand, those who attack faith state that it is all an offshoot of superstitious terror. Psychoanalysis has shown that both these positions are exaggerations. The fact is, that both the anxiety and the beliefs are over-compensations for the Œdipus complex.[1]

Old P. P. Quimby, indeed, who was, up to a certain point, shrewd and in advance of his time, observed that :

" We confound our fears with the thing feared, and place evil in the thing seen or believed . . . We never see what we are afraid of."[2]

It is unfortunate that a church should have been founded upon his work (as has happened to so many prophets) by a person who had so regressed from his liberal views as had Mrs Eddy. In the doctrine of *malicious animal magnetism* (i.e. of black magic), her most repressed anxieties found morbid expression. Her works are replete with such commands as :

" Members will not intentionally or knowingly mentally malpractice . . .
" A member of the Mother Church, who mentally malpractices upon or treats our leader or her staff without her or their consent, shall be disciplined . . .
" If the author of *Science and Health* shall bear witness to the offence of mental malpractice, it shall be considered a sufficient evidence thereof."[3]

[1] " This notion would be hardly worth discussing, in spite of its prevalence, were it not that in the latter instance there is a modicum of truth, there being in fact a close connection between morbid anxiety and most forms of religion. Those who trace morbid anxiety to early religious ideas, however, are guilty of a curiously simple error of logic. Because the two stand in a certain relation to each other, it is inferred that one must be the cause of the other, the truth being that they are both manifestations of a common cause." Jones (E.), " The Pathology of Morbid Anxiety ", *Journal of Abnormal Psychology*, vol. VI. Repub. in his *Papers on Psycho-Analysis* (London, 1923), p. 494.
[2] *Quimby MSS.*, 1861, quoted by Dresser (A. G.), *Philosophy of P. P. Quimby*, p. 90.
[3] Eddy (Mrs M. A. M. B. G. P.), *Church Annual* (Boston, 1924), p. 53.

The same belief in the omnipotence of thought, with a vein of terror of being punished for one's sinful thoughts, troubles the conscience of the other school who inherit the mental condition of Quimby, namely, the New Thought group. Trine fears :

> " The moment we entertain any thoughts of hatred toward another, he gets the effect of those diabolical forces that go out from us."[1]
> " Many a man has been made sick by having the ill thoughts of a number of people centred upon him ; some have been actually killed."[2]

In abstract theory, also, the " New Thoughters " seem to have drifted as far away as did Mrs Eddy from Quimby's flash of insight into the mechanism of fear. Marden asks :

> " What is fear ? It is absolutely nothing. It is a mental illusion. There is no reality behind it. It is to the sane adult what the ghost is to the child."

(There is a spark of truth in this last thought, since behind morbid fears and ghosts alike is the unconscious recollection of the father. But to continue) :

> " There is not a single redeeming feature about fear or any of its numerous progeny. It is always, everywhere, an unmitigated curse."[3]

The title of Marden's book is *Every Man a King*, which signifies that every son is to be equal to his father. Very consistent with this title is the hope (implied by his prediction below) that in the womb-like existence which he thinks of as still in store for the race, anxiety states

---

[1] Trine (R. W.), *In Tune with the Infinite* (London, 1923), p. 70.
[2] Trine (R. W.), *In Tune with the Infinite* (London, 1923), as quoted by Bedgorough (G.), *Harmony or Humbug* (Letchworth, 1917), p. 21.
[3] Bedborough gives p. 26 as his reference, but I have been unable to verify from the edition he used. Of course, in these quotations, the paranoic notion of the *omnipotence of thought* is always involved, seen especially in the following bit of nonsense :—
" A falling state of mind is productive of a falling condition of the body." Trine, *In Tune with the Infinite*, p. 30.

should be absent. Was it, then, his own experience of
Œdipus-begotten anxiety that led him to hope :

> " The coming man will not know fear, which is now the
> greatest enemy of the human race ; for he will not harbour
> the fear thought, which really results from a feeling of
> inefficiency, or inability to cope with the exigencies which
> arise."[1]

It is inconsistent with the paternal origin of conscience
that those things weigh especially heavy upon it which
are closely connected with the father. If, for instance,
we call on the father to witness to the truth of a statement, its gravity before our conscience is increased
beyond all bounds. " Reverence an oath " said Pythagoras and a chorus of other ancient sages and law givers.

Indeed, many sects have always held that such awful
gravity as the oath implied was too dangerous for men
to trifle with at all. Among the Essenes,

> " Any word of theirs had more force than an oath ;
> swearing they avoid, regarding it as worse than perjury,

[1] Marden (O. S.), *Every Man a King*, p. 238.
As we shall in our remaining pages have much to say on auto-
suggestion, it may be worth while to record here a passage from the
most scientific of its contempory exponents, Baudouin. The value of
this excerpt lies in the revelation of connection in Baudoin's case
between fear and repressed death wishes directed against his father.
" One dream," he says, " from far away . . . comes back to me
with singular vividness. . . .
" I have just entered a large bedroom where all three of us sleep. . . .
I stealthily enter, softly opening the door, both from an indefinite
sort of fear and in obedience to instructions.
" My father is there but my father is dead. He is lying . . . in
the iron folding bed. . . . The corpse seemed to me to be in a cage,
a prison. . . . Is this cage-bed my mother's, or is it the one I had
in my earliest childhood . . . with the result that my nightmares
came—horror of horrors ! . . .
" My father is dead, and his body lies imprisoned in that cage of
torture. I am both terrified and delighted. I feel the joy of vengeance.
I have entered for the very purpose of looking at him.
" In my terror I step away from the bed, but on again reaching the
door I am filled with diabolical joy. . . .
" On remembering this dream the following day, I felt horrified
with myself, concealing this imaginary as though it were a real crime.
Never did I relate the incident, but the memory of it remained as genuine
remorse." Baudouin (Ch.), *Birth of Psyche*, transl. Rothwell (London,
1923), pp. 45-8.

for they say that the thing which is not believed without [an appeal to God] stands condemned already."[1]

Exculpating the Father

If we are to show unbounded reverence for the father, however, we must take the further step from which Christian Science has not shrunk, of exonerating him from the blame of having permitted any evil in his universe. The experience of P. P. Quimby with hysteric persons whose physical symptoms so frequently proved to be expressions of their mental twists, suggested to him, as a means of exonerating the father, that all the evil in the world, without exception, should be regarded as mere hysterical mental phenomena. All psychological phenomena were, of course, regarded as conscious and intellectual. Quimby therefore substituted for the old term, Devil, a new term, Error.

" While engaged in his mesmeric experiments, Mr Quimby became more and more convinced·that disease was an error of the mind, not a real thing."[2]

In other words, the more obvious surrogate for the father, namely God, was to be spared all disparaging reflections, by projecting on to him only the most flattering qualities. (Such tendencies to split up the attributes of any object, have long been familiar to psychiatrists.) All disagreeable attributes were to be referred to another surrogate called Error, and then Error was itself to be identified with the sons. Thus we, the sons, are to be responsible for not only our own shortcomings and evil wishes, but for all which exist in this world of the heavenly father's creating :

" According to this new theory, disease is the invention of man. It is caused by a disturbance of the mind—which is spiritual matter—and, therefore, originates there.

[1] *Selections from Josephus*, transl. Thackeray.
[2] Quimby (Geo. A.), in *New England Magazine*, March, 1888. Quoted by Dresser (A. G.), *Philosophy of P. P. Quimby*, p. 15.

" Living in a world full of error in this respect, and educated to believe that disease is something we cannot escape, it is not strange that what we fear comes upon us."[1]

This is the same mechanism as that which Freud postulates as the basis of melancholia. We introject the faults of others into ourselves, as well as vice versa. Flügel tells me[2] of an unhappily married man who became melancholy, and in that state accused himself of faults which everyone could see clearly belonged to his wife. But I return to Quimby, who says :

" Human misery universally arises from some error . . . We confound our fears with the thing feared . . . Here is a great error."[3]

Quimby here is again very close to deep insight. But he also has an extraordinarily materialistic conception of this thing error. He treats of it as though it were a (living ?) *substance*—which is a sort of half-way step toward personifying it as he would have to do if he frankly confessed how far it is a surrogate for unpleasant aspects of the father. He avers :

" A belief makes . . . a man of error, or matter that can be changed."[4]

Change and chance are peculiarly its properties ; it is therefore the negation of law—and the concept of law is derived from that of the judgments of a king or father :

" Truth works by laws, like mathematics ; error like chance."[5]

It will be noted, moreover, that the name with which Quimby re-christened evil, is closely associated with

[1] A patient of Quimby, in *The Advertiser*, Portland, Me., 1862.
[2] In a private conversation in 1925.
[3] *Quimby MSS.*, 1861. Quoted by Dresser (A. G.), *Philosophy of P. P. Quimby*, p. 90.
[4] *Quimby MSS.*, 1861. Dresser (A. G.), *Philosophy of P. P. Quimby*, p. 108.
[5] *Quimby MSS.* Dresser (H. W.), *The Quimby Manuscripts* (N. Y.), p. 181.

the question of knowledge—a question which essentially means, to the child, sexual knowledge.

It is thought at the moment that Quimby said : " The father does no evil. Evil is something due to the son ", a part of Quimby's unconscious substituted in place of *something*, this word *error*, which was to imply " really it is all due to father after all, because it is he who does secret things [with mother] about which they deceive us poor children ! "

My hypothesis receives confirmation when we find Quimby, after this analysis of evil, resolving upon the formulation of a *science* as a means of cure. Sciences, it is generally conceded, spring essentially from the impulse of curiosity, which has in turn been largely resolved by psycho-analysis into a by-product of infantile *voyeurism* concerned with what the parents do together to make a baby. Moreover, Quimby expressly calls his new science, the science *of life*, and in the same breath equates error to the opposite of life and birth, namely death :

> " The science of life is to know how to keep man from getting into death or error. This is my theory : to put man in possession of a science that will destroy the ideas of the sick, and teach man . . . life free from error."[1]
> " As science is light, it . . . like the sun burns up the darkness of error . . .
> " Matter to *God or Science* is a medium of communication."[2]

The term, Science, occurs very frequently. It obviously represents something very central in his psyche :

> " I am often asked what I call my cures. I answer, the effect of a science, because I know how I do them."[3]

---

[1] *Quimby MSS.*, March, 1861.   Quoted by Dresser (A. G.), *Philosophy of P. P. Quimby*, pp. 103-4.
[2] *Quimby MSS.*, Dresser (H. W.), *Quimby MSS.* (New York), p. 408. (Italics mine).
[3] *Quimby MSS.*, May, 1861.   Quoted by Dresser (A. G.), *Philosophy of P. P. Quimby*, p. 79.   Also quoted by Dresser (H. W.), *The Quimby MSS.*, p. 286.

Naturally Quimby's pupil, Mrs Eddy, became impressed with this noun, which, as we know, she wove into the name of the cult she organized. She glorifies the term—a glorification, really, of the father, for we shall elsewhere find her equating the terms Science and God as Quimby has done above—at the expense of two rival cults being popularized by women leaders :

" Science is not susceptible of being held as a mere theory. It is hoary with time. It takes hold of eternity, voices the infinite, and governs the universe. No greater opposites can be conceived of, physically, morally and spiritually, than Christian Science, Spiritualism, and Theosophy . . .

" Theosophy is no more allied to Christian Science than the odour of the upas tree is to the sweet breath of Spring-tide, or the brilliant coruscations of the northern sky are to solar heat and light."[1]

In his turn Emile Coué also came to inherit the enthusiasm of Quimby for an exact formulation of suggestive therapy :

" M Coué went to Nancy and by 1910 had moulded his study into a complete and exact science . . . His work at first was confined to Lorraine peasants, for whose simple minds his theories needed no explanation ; but as M Coué's teaching has spread more widely, further explanation has been deemed necessary."[2]

Another sentiment of Quimby's which was adopted by Mrs Eddy was his solicitude lest the father be blamed for any of the evil of the world. She formulated it ascetically for the new religion :

" Sorrow is salutary . . . Trials are proof of God's care."

She similarly took over Quimby's accent upon the magical importance of truthfulness combined with the attribution of the source of evil to the sons and never to the father.

" If anyone is untruthful, his mental state weighs against

[1] Eddy (Mrs M. A. M. B. P. G.), *No and Yes* (Boston, 1918), pp. 13-4.
[2] Lady Noble of Ardkinglas : *M. Coué and Auto-Suggestion* (Chatham and London, 1924), p. 3.

his healing power; and similar effects come from pride, envy, lust and all fleshly vices."[1]

More notably still did Mrs Eddy make the term, *error*, a key-word in Christian Science. There, as I have intimated, it replaced the earlier Christian concept of a personal devil, because it is a more effective repression, through being de-personalized, of the seamy side of the father's character. Error would seem to represent fundamentally the *deceitfulness of the father*, who does not tell his children about his sexual agressions against the mother.

In most religions where God is strongly emphasized as the embodiment of all good, his opposite, Tiamet, Ahriman, Satan, the Flesh, etc., is pictured in contrast. In other words the purely lovable qualities of the father-image cannot easily be idealized save by splitting the actual image into two. We then have one image representing all that was loved or admired in the father, the other, all that was hated in him.

But in certain religions, the evil half of the father-*imago* (doubtless because apprehended as being what it truly is) is repressed by the excessive conscience. Even the devil must not remain to challenge the perfection of the father. God is good, and good is *all*.

But we know that to wipe any concept out of existence is not so easy. What is repressed is for ever attempting to come back, assuming newer and newer disguises to pass the censor. Thus, in these religions which refuse to admit any kind of devil, we get such statements as that evil is the reverse side, or the absence, or the denial, of good. Or the devil is projected on to man himself, who becomes the one corrupting factor in a universe which was made perfect, as in the words of the familiar hymn :

> " Where every prospect pleases,
> And only man is vile."

[1] Eddy (Mrs M. A. M. B. G. P.), *Rudimentary Divine Science* (Boston, 1918), p. 9.

In the case of Christian Science, then, the attributes of Satan have been projected on to man-made Error.

But New Thought, as well as Christian Science, took from Quimby the idea, that all misfortune is the fault of the son who has rejected his father :

> " Man is the only one who has to do with evil ; he alone is its author. Man, who in his thought separates himself from Divine Being, in whom alone true happiness and blessedness can be found."[1]

Evil wishes (the first of which in a male infant are regularly directed against the father) are considered positive things ; and Trine thus rehabilitates the technique of sorcery :

> " In the degree that we hold a person in the thought of evil or error, do we suggest evil or error to him . . . And so in this way we may be sharers in the very evil-doing in which we hold another in thought."[2]

Sthenicism

The exercises of various sthenic cults, however much they may be rationalized as being simply intended for the physical, intellectual, emotional or conative benefit of those practising them, often are so severe that we must suspect them of a self punitive motive.

These movements will be the more easily understood if we consider how frequently religious cults which make a point of the perfecting of the individual or of his advancement along a " mystic path ", employ practices of an exceedingly painful nature. That these are a form of self punishment for Œdipus wishes, seems inferable from the combination of these exercises with the purpose of reunion with the heavenly father, as in Christian penances before Communion. Among those Moham-medan Sufis known as Dervishes :

> " The Sa'dites, Rifaites and Ahmadites have peculiar feats, peculiar to each *tarika*, of eating glowing embers

[1] Trine (R. W.), *Greatest Thing Ever Known* (London, 1898), p. 8.
[2] Trine (R. W.), *In Tune with the Infinite* (London, 1923), p. 71.

and live serpents, or scorpions and glass, of passing needles through their bodies and spikes into their eyes . . . Such exhibitions . . . may in part be tricks and in part rendered possible by a hypnotic state."[1]

Both the self punishment motive and desire for mystical union with the father were apparent in a Dervish ceremony at Kairoan, holy city of North Africa, which the writer, with a friend, Mr Robbins, attended and took careful notes of. These notes were too long to include here, but may be summarized.

I counted 110 Dervishes taking part in the exercises. Behind a grille at my right were some of their women. The priests chanted certain refrains over and over, and at certain times the assembly joined in or swayed together rhythmically. Prayers, choruses and announcements followed, the latter sometimes answered by shrill cries from the women. A line of men standing at the rear did a special swaying exercise which seemed a sort of warming up.

From this line individuals presently leaped into the middle of the room, and there ducked and waved most wildly to the sound of drums and tambourines. Their facial expressions at this time were often most sensual.

Apparently this induced anæsthesia. Some of these men then leaped rhythmically about the mosque like frogs, while pressing weapons against their bodies. Others had weights of eight pounds or more affixed to the skin of breast and shoulders by hooks. Others allowed pointed iron weapons to be thrust through the flesh towards their entrails. Others eagerly ate the spiny fronds of cactus. One held a live scorpion over his mouth and with great gusto snapped his teeth on to it and ate it down. Other like things were done, but I have described only what I was close enough to inspect and be reasonably sure there was no fraud about.

In all these cases there seemed to be at the time neither bleeding nor any facial indications of pain. Apparently

[1] McDonald (D. B.), in art. " Dervishes " in *Encyclopædia of Islam*.

L

the priests administered no ordeal until satisfied that the candidate had worked himself into a sufficiently ecstatic condition to be insensible to pain. The sense of union with the father apparently anticipated the self-punishment that followed it.

At the Gurdiev Institute for Harmonic Development of man, which is based upon Dervish principles, the dance is made a leading feature. Whatever motives of self-punishment, or of other expressions of attitude connected with the father, inspire the Sufi ceremonies, may be presumed to be present in some degree in the Gurdievian ones developed therefrom. But the religious aspect begins to be relegated to the background, and the alleged benefit to the participant is paramount.

By these dances, the reader must not understand anything in the way of ballroom gyrations. They are series of special bodily postures gone through successively in time to music. But my saying this gives the reader no impression of their extreme difficulty. Each motion of right or left arm or leg or of the head has to be made on a certain count, independently of every other. Thus no " dance " can become as mechanical a routine as is ordinarily the case. One has to keep his mind on what he is doing, every moment ; and if once he becomes confused, it is all up with him. These dances, at the time the present writer was visiting the institute, were done very late at night, after a long day of gruelling physical labour.[1]

---

[1] There were also special dances for nearly every individual. The postures were such as one wouldn't ordinarily assume. This was to get us out of the limited repertory of physical positions which is said by Gurdiev to characterize each person ordinarily. Some students told me that they had experienced indescribably new emotional effects. Others denied this.

Particularly interesting is the " ' stop '-exercise ". The students start running across the hall. Suddenly Gurdiev cries " Stop " ! Instantly every one must " freeze " in whatever attitude he happens to be in. Each tries also to arrest his train of thoughts. He then notes what he had been thinking and feeling, and what are the positions and tensions in every part of his body, systematically examined—his repertoire of typical attitudes.

Some Dervish performances such as these we have mentioned exceed in their self-punitive zeal anything likely to be common in purely secular sthenic movements. We sometimes see the severity of their ordeals approached, however, by certain physical culturists. Self-punishment as well as desire for fame may well be a motive in channel swims, prize-fighting and wrestling, Marathon runs, six-day bicycle races, etc.

In this chapter, then, we have seen how the father's voice, in conscience, made even some socialists as humble as monks, and held Kenyon back from giving any movement his whole-hearted support. In the religiously inclined, respect for the father motivated a search for some conception such as Devil or Error, upon which evil could be blamed, and it at times led to self-punishment.

CHAPTER II

PERSECUTING THE SONS

INTRODUCTORY REMARKS

THE anxiety not to betray hatred of the father and sympathy with the rebellious sons may lead one to displace the outward acts of hatred on to the sons, and actually to persecute them. This conduct is, of course, facilitated by the presence of a masochistic type of affect which finds expression in identification of oneself with the sons.

The individual who is thus strongly reacting against his impulses to rebellion, may be at pains to simulate an exaggerated regard for authority.

If he is tempted inwardly to mock at his father, or, expressing this tendency in sublimated form, to blaspheme God, his over-compensation causes him to wage war upon blasphemers and to pass laws against them.

As the demand of the son is naturally for equalization, it follows that wherever we find a strong protest against this tendency on the part of those whose general attitude is revolutionary, we are entitled to suspect that this is an over-compensation.

The child is unable to compete with his father, except at a disadvantage. Therefore the father has little to fear from competition ; and may advantageously exploit this principle between members of the family as a means both of increasing the collective income and also of preventing combination against himself. This will usually be resented by the sons. But they may react against their own resentment and espouse the father's game.

We have already considered how the feelings directed against one's father may very easily be displaced on to one's son. In the material we have here to treat, it is peculiarly difficult to distinguish between what is so motivated, and what is the result of hatred of the sons begotten of genuine love of the fathers. When St Paul was zealously persecuting the Christians, this must have seemed a real hatred of this rebellious new sect ; a hatred apparently based upon love of Yaveh and his priesthood. But, we are told, all the time St Paul was " kicking against the pricks ", i.e. his persecuting activities were but a reaction-formation against a secret sympathy with the young sect ; a sympathy so strong that presently it overmastered his repressions and converted him (return of the repressed). The fact is noteworthy, that this conversion was accompanied by temporary blindness (symbolic castration).

For this reason it seems necessary here to handle simultaneously the material on persecution out of reaction-formation, together with that of true son-hatred.

The harshness of ceremonies of initiation among savages, together with such symbolic castration features as the knocking out or filing away of teeth, almost compel us to recognize that the jealousy of the fathers is here finding a culminating expression.[1] It is as though vengeance were being taken, and an old score being settled.[2]

The assumed need of keeping the sons from entering too easily into the group of the fathers was one motive

---

[1] Reik, Dr. Th. : " Pubertätsriten Der Wilden," *Probleme der Religionspsychologie*, pp. 59 ff.

[2] " In the cruel rites which are so often inflicted on the novices by the elder members of the community it is possible to see a manifestation of that fear and hatred which fathers often feel towards their sons and which mothers often feel towards their daughters —feelings which often correspond in nature and intensity to the equivalent emotions in the children themselves . . . the pretended killing or death of the novice being frequently of the nature of a punishment on the talion principle for the thoughts of patricide or matricide which the children may themselves have entertained towards their parents." Flügel (J. C.), *Psycho-Analytic Study of the Family*, 1923, pp. 83-4.

behind initiation ceremonies. As carried out among savages, the harshness of these doubtless is of a real utility in weaning the boy away from too great fixation on his mother, by their emphasis, reinforced by powerful effects, on the principle that the victim is being reborn.

The barbarisms of primitive initiation have their echo in those of modern secret societies, where the tendency to inflict suffering becomes subject to civilized repression, and survives only in such feeble degree as can mask under the participants' sense of humour.[1]

Occasionally the tide of hostility to the sons which these initiations represent, becomes too strong for the repressions, and shows its real intensity in the actual maiming or killing of candidates.

This is most apt to be the case where the initiators are still but little removed from primitivism, or, what primitivism really means, from infantilism. That is, the younger the father group itself is, the more atrociously is it likely to treat its (still younger) " sons ". In the U.S.A. these conditions are sometimes found in college, and frequently in high school, Greek-letter fraternities. In the college fraternities the youth of the members is partially offset by their being a more cultured group than the average citizenry. But the high school fraternities of the United States are such a menace that they have largely had to be broken up by State legislation.

Parenthetically, we may note that the above facts in regard to high schools show the purely relative nature of any division of persons according to age into a father group and a son group. The Œdipus complex is the same whether manifested towards a " father " or toward a " son "; circumstances determine which terms we shall apply to the respective persons in a relationship. The initiators to the high school societies may next year become candidates for a college fraternity; those who will then initiate them will feel as sons to fathers with

---

[1] For a summary of the grotesqueries of these associations see *The Nation* (New York, 1925). Also *Labour Age* (New York, 1925).

respect to their college tutors and lecturers ; these will feel in a like position relatively to the older members of the professorial board, and so on.

ECONOMICO-POLITICAL TYPE

A complaint is often voiced, that social reformers ought to appeal to the altruism and enlightened self-interest of the upper class, instead of to the self-protective instincts, the greed and the jealousy of the submerged. To this, socialists have been able to reply that the earliest socialists took just this course, but that it got them nowhere. To-day, some employers are beginning to take a more generous attitude, and it is one of the possibilities of the future, that appeals by the workers to their employer's better side may be less unfruitful than they have been in the past, and than sole reliance upon the machinery of coercion (unions). But, of course, the attitude of the worker himself is influenced by the Œdipus Complex quite as much as is that of the capitalist. Strikes are not so purely as they are assumed to be the result of calculation of expediency, any more than are all acts of discipline or reduction of wages.

Failure to take into account this fact leads to those bitter accusations of one another's good faith, which are often heard. In connection with an instance to be cited, let me recall to the reader the well-known fact that almost any popular cause has its list of devotees who have been willing to suffer and die for it. Socialism, Anarchism and Syndicalism are only a few of those which have made a calendar like that which the Catholic Church made, of their heroic leaders who unflinchingly went to prison or faced a lynching mob. To say, therefore, as does Hilaire Belloc, that :

" No word ending in ' ism ' ever made a martyr or an apostle or a hero or a saint."[1]

[1] Belloc (Hilaire), *Economics For Helen* (New York, 1924), p. 123.

is to add insult to the injury of the infamous persecutions such as the fathers have carried on against the sons from time immemorial, and carry on to-day from Hungary[1] in the East to California[2] in the West. Indeed, a

[1] " The arrival in Budapest, and . . . arrest, of a former member of the Soviet Government of Hungary, has been the signal for a period of police terror in that city unequalled since Horthy's bloody repression of the Soviet Government in 1919.

" News of subsequent events were hidden behind a veil of silence which fell over Budapest, and which was only lifted by the Vienna Press during the week-end. All last week the news agencies gave absolutely no information as to the terrible scenes which were being enacted.

" Altogether it appears nearly 100 persons, among them a number of women, were arrested as suspected Communists. They were subjected by the police, in effort to extract information, to fearful brutalities.

" Floggings and batterings with cudgels were administered unmercifully. Rakosi is reported to have had his finger-nails torn off and to have been tortured with burning embers. The beatings have seriously injured his spine. The women prisoners were not spared. One in particular, Frau Hamann, is suffering from terrible injuries.

" While all this was going on, the police building was heavily guarded by a cordon of police. . . . The representatives of . . . newspapers, who usually visit the police headquarters every day for news were refused admission.

" In the streets around the building terrible cries of pain were heard by horror-stricken passers-by. Even the bourgeois papers comment on these proceedings as ' a dark reminder ' of the early days of the Horthy regime."

The present writer can testify to having seen the welts on the backs of working men where they had just been beaten in Budapest by the police, out of pure malice.

[2] " A short report on conditions during 1924 in the United States has just been issued by the American Civil Liberties' Union. Fewer free speech prosecutions, police interference with meetings and cases of mob violence have been reported than in any year since the beginning of the war. And yet in 1925, the report shows, there were 233 persecutions involving freedom of speech or assembly, 41 cases of mob violence, and 16 lynchings of Negroes. Mob violence centred chiefly about the Klu Klux Klan, but ' the violence was more often against the Klan than by it, as in previous years '. California led the country in the number of prosecutions, with 202 persons, all members of the I.W.W., arrested under the criminal syndicalism act. In West Virginia, thousands of evictions took place in the strike of the coal miners, but the old cases against United Mine Workers' officials in connection with the armed march in 1921, were dropped. Three important court decisions are listed in the report as affecting civil rights :—

" (1) The decision of the Californian Supreme Court, upholding the Busick injunction, which prohibits membership in the I.W.W.

" (2) The U.S. Supreme Court decision upholding the Clayton Act provision granting jury trials in cases of criminal contempt growing out of labour disputes. and

" (3) The nullification by the Oregon Supreme Court of the law compelling attendance at public schools, instead of parochial schools."
The World To-morrow (New York, March, 1925).

pamphlet just issued, giving details of conditions in Italy, Poland, Germany, India, Hungary, Spain, Japan, Esthonia, Bulgaria, Roumania, Venezuela and Russia, opens with the statement that :

"Throughout the world to-day more prisoners are now serving terms for their political and industrial beliefs and activities than at any time in recorded history."[1]

So fierce is the persecution of the rebellious sons that :

"In some countries . . . there are fewer political prisoners for the simple . . . reason that the party in power shot them instead of locking them up."[2]

We have previously told how limitations on freedom of speech are resented by rebels as being somehow a castration of them. But where a reaction-formation has set in against rebel tendencies, we shall expect to find persecution of the sons connived at. In the typical radical baiter, it is difficult to know whether his attitude is due to reaction against father-hatred, by displacement on to the sons, or to a direct love of the father and consequent hatred of rebellious sons. Either motive is effective toward the objective of cutting off their speech.

An illustrative case was reported in The New York Nation.[2] A meeting at Wilkes Barre, Penn., was ended by American Legionaries marching in, armed with bayonets, and "breaking it up at the point of their guns". Mayor D. N. Hart, far from protecting the wronged parties, chose to champion the strong against the weak :

"I shall not tolerate any organization holding meetings in this community that is opposed by the American Legion. All meetings of this character in future will be submitted to the Legion for approval before they are permitted.

[1] *Political Persecution To-day*, published by International Committee for Political Prisoners (Chairman, Baldwin, R. N.).
[2] February 13th, 1924.

Freedom of speech under the American flag is welcome, but under the red flag of anarchy will never be tolerated."[1]

I choose this instance because the language used by the Mayor is that appropriate not to the oppressing father but to an oppressed son. One would think the mayor and the Legion were the ones being outraged. In short, we have here once more the interesting mechanism of a transportation of rôles, i.e. the introjection on to the subject himself and those identified with him, of the affects which belong in reality to the object.

Without venturing on to the controversial ground of their desirability or otherwise, any well-informed person must grant that the number of considerable syndicalist as well as democratic producer-co-operative ventures

[1] Similar cases are so numerous, that to go into them all would be clearly impossible. I may, however, be pardoned for briefly describing one instance of which I have personal knowledge. In May, 1923, while a strike was in progress in Los Angeles Harbour, Upton Sinclair and his brother-in-law, Hunter Kimborough, chanced to be in the office of J. H. Price, President of the Merchants and Manufacturers' Association. They heard Hammond, of the Hammond Lumber Co., demand of Price that the Dock Strike should be broken, and heard Price assure him that it should be done without delay. Next morning the police of Los Angeles Harbour threw into jail 500 men who were merely listening to speakers on " Freedom Hill ", a vacant lot owned by a sympathiser. On hearing of this, Sinclair and a score of respectably dressed friends called on Mayor Cryer, of Los Angeles. They extracted from him a promise to telephone the Chief of Police, Oakes, at the Harbour that he should protect them in their right to free speech. Several then drove to the harbour, called on the chief, and notified him that we would read the American Constitution to the strikers on the hill.

Chief Oakes asserted : " You're not going up there to break the law." " Break what law ? " asked the writer. " We'll tell you the law when we arrest you," replied the Chief of Police.

In the evening a cordon of police were at the foot of the hill and another on its crest. These kept everyone away except Sinclair's party, so that the speakers addressed only ranks of policemen. Four in succession stood up, and after saying a dozen words, on the right of free speech, each was arrested, charged with " suspicion of criminal syndicalism ". They were kept in jail until next afternoon, and their requests to inform their wives where they were, or to communicate with their lawyers, were refused. They then got out on bail. The charge against them was changed to that of blocking traffic, and " uttering certain thoughts and theories " likely to excite violence, " in contempt of the constitution ". In court, later, the case was dismissed. Naturally, the case resulted in hundreds of members being recruited for the local branch of the Civil Liberties' Union.

which are succeeding economically, from Scandinavia in the north to Italy in the south of Europe, is extremely large. And the second of these movements, the co-operative, is at last getting a foothold in America.[1] Taking this into consideration as well as the socialism prevalent among primitive peoples, we must expect a hidden complex in a writer like Hilaire Belloc. Only so would he be likely, without qualification nor defining his terms, to echo the opinion that

> " Socialism never has been put into practice, and never can be put into practice. There have been attempts at it, but even when they are sincere and not the mere product of alien despotism, they break down."[2]

But by this stroke of the pen, Belloc symbolically wipes out of existence all those groups who have ever rebelled successfully against the institution of property— one which essentially represents the father. That is, he wipes out revolutionary sons. That this represents a wish fulfilment in his case, seems to be evidenced by the general hostility of this writer to almost every single one of the social movements which we shall herein find to represent sons as against fathers.

HUMANITARIAN TYPE

We have seen what becomes of some of the cruel tendencies towards sons, to which civilized society denies the adequate expression of savage initiations. These passions, suppressed, do not

> " Fold their tents like the Arabs
> And as silently steal away."

---

[1] If we modify still more our definition of Socialism, so as to include the Rochdale type of co-operatives, we have a movement which is enormous and successful in Europe.

[2] Belloc (Hilaire), *Economics For Helen* (New York, 1924), p. 125.

There is evidence, rather, that they largely find their outlet through certain alternative channels.

For members of superior groups one such channel is the maltreatment of members of inferior groups. This may be said to have three aspects. (a) Advanced nations like Great Britain, Holland, Japan and the United States, massacre the more primitive Hindoos, Javanese, Koreans or Haitians. (b) Social classes privileged because of rank, property, profession, or intellectual or moral virtue ostracize, starve, exploit, or brutally punish classes handicapped by inferiority-tradition, lack of training, poverty or criminal tendency. (c) Members of honoured or highly evolved races humiliate and torture members of despised or child-like races. I am disposed to maintain in the discussion below, that in humanitarian efforts we have largely a reaction-formation against the tendencies manifested in these three forms of son-persecution.

Massacre of Child-like Peoples by Civilized

Cases of (a) are pretty well aired in the public press. British readers get very mild reports of the harsher features of their own rule in India, or their action against strikers in China, and are led to believe that these were justified ; but they may get a moderately good account of American terrorism in Panama, Nicaragua, Haiti, Santo Domingo, etc. Americans similarly hear nothing of the methods of their marines in these last places, or else are convinced that they were provoked by natives' aggressions ; but their press keeps them fairly well informed of the injustices committed by Great Britain, Japan and others.

And so on. Except as regards each reader's own country, the facts will not be unfamiliar. The exact truth, in most cases, is difficult to sift from conflicting reports. It may also be alleged that, as the peoples at home keep imperfectly informed of what is being done abroad by their agents, no responsibility rests with them.[1] But are we to assume that this persistence in ignorance is unconnected with repressed desìres ? The whole of Freud's *Psycho-Pathology of Everyday Life* is an argument that almost nothing in our conduct is wholly unwished for by us.

I shall not go at length here into the matter of the complaisance of the people at home. But the mutual support given by governments to one another in these situations, indicates that at any rate the officials comprising them are class-conscious, all being fathers who must stand together against rebellious sons.

My point is illustrated by the report of a bit of uncalled-for inhumanity in connection with Spain's recent struggle with Abd el Krim :

> " The British Government has refused to allow the International Red Cross to take medical supplies to these parts because the Spanish Government refused to regard these people as belligerents. It says they are rebels, and rebels shall have no resource to International Law. . . . No Power has applied to the British and Spanish Governments to prevent the import of guns and ammunition which, as a matter of fact, are going through the Spanish lines. It is the Red Cross supplies that it is difficult to get through."[2]

In America, where the cult of Father Militarism is young, but exceedingly vigorous since we made war to suppress it in Germany, one of its best exponents is doughty old Hudson Maxim, who believes :

> " No branch of education—not even hygiene, moral reform, cleanliness, temperance, and right living—would be so influential for betterment as would the introduction of the Swiss system of military training."[3]

---

[1] And indeed the British Labour Party, and Socialists, and their affiliates in the United States, have opposed the imperialism of their governments. But in the recent Moroccan crisis the French Socialists (Communists, to their credit, apart), vacillated pitifully.

[2] Burns (C. De Lisle), " Christian Nations and Others ", *The Monthly Record of South Place Ethical Society* (London, June, 1925), p. 7.

[3] Maxim (Hudson), *Defenceless America* (London, New York and Toronto), p. 291.

The principle on which officials seem to act was thus callously but frankly expressed by this American arch-militarist, who believes the heavenly father is with him :

" There are times when throats have to be cut, and when God is on the side of the executioner."[1]

This writer apparently believes that in every person the belligerent motives are invariably the strongest ones.[2]

[1] Maxim (Hudson), *Defenceless America* (London, New York and Toronto), p. 282.

[2] Regarding war as an expression of sinister psychological trends, Ernest Jones is very pessimistic concerning human ability to control this phenomenon. His reasons for believing that wars are bound to recur periodically as the result of accumulated tensions deserve to be quoted :—
" The question arises whether there is not in the human mind some . . . set of recurrently acting agents which tends to . . . find or create pretexts for wars whatever the external situation may be [and] that man cannot live for more than a certain period without indulging his warlike impulses. . . . Another possibility . . . is that man tends to prefer the solution of various socio-political problems by means of war to their solution in any other way . . . it might be very plausibly argued that what happens historically is a periodic outburst of warlike impulses followed by a revulsion against war . . . which is again succeeded by a forgetting of the horrors involved and a gradually accumulating tension that once more leads to an explosion." Jones (E.), *War and Individual Psychology*, published in the *Sociological Review*, 1905, vol. VIII, p. 167. Republished in his *Essays in Applied Psycho-Analysis*, 1923, p. 368.
Again : " The influence of social situations is very apt to be in . . . the direction of undoing the effects of sublimation, thus leading to the adoption of a lower or more primitive standard of behaviour. . . . Sublimations are mainly individual creations, whereas the unconscious repressed impulses are more uniformly and generally distributed ; a relapse therefore takes place in the direction of the greatest common measure of the whole. . . . Most committees will display types of behaviour involving perhaps injustice, meanness, inconsiderateness and lack of responsibility of a kind that would be disavowed by any single member acting independently. The blood-thirsty and often indiscriminate cruelty of mobs is notorious. . . . This massive social contact creates none of these impulses ; it only releases them. . . .
" Every nation whole-heartedly maintains the view that it was forced to go to war, regretfully and entirely against its will, by the wicked machinations of some other nation. Now this is just the attitude which in private life we see adopted towards any anti-social act. . . . The person concerned makes every endeavour to shift his guilt of responsibility on to others or on to circumstances, and seeks to defend his conduct under cover of all imaginable excuses, pretexts, rational-izations." Jones (E.), *op. cit.*, pp. 370-1.

In war the old men stay at home with the women, while their sons are sent forth to be punished or killed. Such a statement may sound cynical, but the facts appear to be in keeping with the demands of the Œdipus complex. Leagues of youth are largely pacifist in every country in the world ; I am not aware of any centenarians' clubs which have so recorded themselves. That, as Dr M. D. Eder perceives :

" This jealousy of the fathers toward their male children, unconscious in part or wholly so, is one of the causes of war, seems not to have escaped the notice of the youth of this age—at least of some of the more sensitive among them, poets and novelists. War, with its special death roll among the young fulfils the desire of the old men for the removal of their lusty rivals ; the war memorials, the cenotaphs are not only monuments raised in expiation of the old people's sins, but are also survivals of days when it was feared that the ghosts of the killed, taking material shape, would revenge themselves on the living ; these monumental erections will prevent the dead arising."[1]

Here then, at least, would seem to be a case of humanitarianism receiving impetus from reaction against the father's persecuting attitude.

Graybeards from the earliest times have made light of all hopes of eventually abolishing war. Plato said .

" All states are in a perpetual war with all. For that which we call peace is no more than a name, whilst in reality Nature has set all communities in an unproclaimed but everlasting war against each other."[2]

" General " Homer Lea sees the partial truth (for the word *only* might better have been omitted) that

" Nations are only Man in the aggregate of his deceptions and crimes and depravity ; and, so long as these constitute the basis of individual impulse so long will they control the acts of nations."

[1] Eder (M. D.), " Psycho-Analysis in Politics ", in *Social Aspects of Psycho-Analysis*, ed. by E. Jones (London, 1924), pp. 143-4.
[2] Plato, as quoted by Maxim (H.).

Overlooking any possibility of the masses (sons) refusing obedience to their governments (fathers) when these call upon the people to endure again the increasing frightfulness of modern war, or any possibility of an international police (neutral brotherhood) being substituted for national armies (partizan hatred) " General " Lea concludes that

> " Only when arbitration is able to unravel the tangled skein of crime and hypocrisy among individuals can it be extended to communities and nations. . . .
> " When, therefore, the merchant arbitrates with the customer he is about to cheat ; when trusts arbitrate with the people they are about to fleece ; when the bulls and the bears arbitrate with the lambs they are about to shear ; when the thief arbitrates with the man he is about to rob, or the murderer with his victim, and so on throughout the category of crime, then will communities be able to dispense with laws, and international thievery and deception, cheating and murder, resort to arbitration."[1]

Some learned father-types indeed—and those not all Germans like Treitschke—express a seeming dread of peace, exclaiming :

> " Universal peace appears less as a dream than as a nightmare ! "[2]

Victimization of the Wicked and the Economically Weak by the Good and Strong

The literature of social revolt teems with citations of injustice by ruling classes. Karl Marx's *Das Kapital* is full of them. They are what give revolt its power. Where they are inflicted upon a large group, or one able to fight back, the particular situation brings its own remedy. The sinister motive, however, remains ; too often it wreaks itself on those groups which are least

---

[1] Lea (Gen. [Sic.] Homer), as approvingly quoted by Maxim. *Defenceless America* (London, New York and Toronto), p. 33.
[2] " A nightmare which shall be realised only when the ice has crept to the heart of the sun." Cramb (Prof. J. A.), *Origins and Destiny of Imperial Britain.* Quoted by Maxim (H.), *Defenceless America,* p. 41.

able to organize themselves and must await the tardy chivalry of public enlightenment.

I have in mind particularly the conditions in our prisons. A few " model " ones serve the public as an excuse for pretending all is well. But many prisons are places where, under the excuse of protecting society, sadists employed as jailers (fathers) wreck upon mentally and morally stunted persons (sons) the Œdipus complex of the law-abiding community (fathers).

All that has been said applies also to punishments in the army and navy, where surrogates for father or son respectively are found in officer or man. Especially apparent is the relationship where the offender is youthful. Such punishments attain a harshness going beyond the needs of the situation. They therefore substantiate my hypothesis of a hatred which arises out of unresolved personal conflicts such as Sadism or the Œdipus complex or a combination of both seem alone adequate to explain. This is borne out by such accounts as the following :

" My life as a naval rating during the late war impressed upon me the brutalizing effect of such a life, not only on combatants . . . but upon everyone remotely connected with war, and the training (commencing at the public schools) for war . . .

" For trivial offences such as smoking or returning late from leave, etc., boys are strapped down and lashed with a cane, as many as nine and twelve strokes being given, the terrible pain and shock often causing fainting and making any kind of movement extremely painful for days, the weals often breaking and discharging blood and matter. This punishment can be used *ad lib.*, as no returns are required to be kept.

" Even this sickening brutality is excelled by a birching, which punishment was revived in 1917."[1]

---

[1] " Before undergoing this ordeal the young victim is medically examined to see if his heart, etc., are fit. The victim is stripped below the waist and laid across a whipping horse, and his ankles and wrists secured with cords, drawing his extremities close down to the deck. A petty officer then advances, armed with a formidable instrument resembling a collection of long knotted wires, and lays on the first stroke with all his might, when an attendant officer calls ' One '. Slowly

M

This account is contained in a pacifist publication—
that is to say, by an organ of those who are in revolt
against the father as seen in ruthless imperialism such
as has been previously touched on.

Cruelty to the Base-Born on the part of the Nobly-Born

The English-speaking peoples seem more deficient
than most others in capacity to get along on friendly
terms with the more child-like races. This shows itself
in (a) the stricter tabu maintained by the average
member of this race against intermarriage, and his related phobia of " contamination " (jealousy of imagined
superior potency)[1] by mere presence at the same table,
or under the same roof, of a " coloured " person, (b) in
the way that those among whom he lives hate the
" Anglo-Saxon " for his arrogance, and (c) in the United
States, the retrogression to Lynch Law.[2]

the cruelty continues until twelve strokes have been given, by which
time the delicate white skin is a mass of weals and bloody lacerations,
and the poor lad's mental and physical condition can only be dimly
imagined. The first man now retires, and a second, armed with a
fresh birch, takes his place. At the end of the twenty-four strokes
(which is generally interrupted by swooning) the terrible object left
gasping and sobbing with eyes starting from their sockets and blood
and bits of broken birch everywhere, bears but little resemblance to
anything human. He is taken to sick-bay, where his lacerations are
dressed, causing further exquisite anguish. He is detained there for
twelve hours, until his dangerous phyiscal and mental disturbance has
passed." May (J. Hooper), " Brutality in the Navy," in *No More
War* (London, September, 1924).

For an account of old time punishments in the Navy and flogging
around the fleet, see Clowes (W. Laird) *The Royal Navy*, London, 1900.
vol. V, pp. 26 *et seq.*

[1] In dreams of women the black regularly stands for potency, says
E. Jones (verbal communication to the writer).

[2] I shall only treat of the last point, as the others mainly involve
motives which we are not here considering. Even in the last point
one other motive, namely Sadism, admittedly plays perhaps the pre-
dominant part. It is hard to disentangle this motive from the Oedipus
complex. As there are two great nationalities involved in Anglo-
Saxondom, let me give one citation concerning each. The first is
about justice in the district of Kenya :—

" Within the last year or two there has been a recrudescence of
certain very disagreeable signs of cruelty. In 1920, and immediately
after the war, it might be said that the situation was so unsettled that,
naturally, crimes of violence would occur in the relationship between
the blacks and whites in Africa, but in 1923 a rather alarming case

In America, lynching is oftenest meted out for a real or alleged sexual offence (using the word sexual in its popular, restricted sense). This fact alone links it up strongly with the Oedipus complex. But statistics show that upon the whole negroes are not, as is pretended, more often guilty of such offence than whites, but less often. Yet they are oftener lynched.

The quotation deals with the revolting punishment of a negro woman for the

"remark that if she knew the names of the persons who lynched her husband the Saturday before, she would have them prosecuted. This was her offence—for this she was lynched."

Note below the juxtaposition of " agony " in the victim and " glee " in the mob.

"At the time she was lynched, Mary Turner was in her eighth month of pregnancy. . . . Her ankles were tied together, and she was tied to the tree head downward. Gasoline from the automobiles was thrown on her clothing, and while she writhed in agony and the mob howled in glee,

occurred in the Colony of Kenya, in which an Englishman, who was a landowner and employer of labour in the Colony, began to flog a native and forced other natives to continue the flogging. Eventually the native died. The case in itself was sufficiently astonishing, but— what is far more important for us—cases of cruelty occur wherever there is an immense amount of power in the hands of the few and no power at all in the hands of the many. We have innumerable instances of the same kind in past history under slavery. We find them as far back as Roman times and before, and in recent times in nearly all parts of the world. A few come to our notice.

" Such instances of cruelty are significant, but the effect they produce on the administration of justice is more important. In the case of murder by flogging in Kenya, a jury of Englishmen acquitted the white employer of anything more than bodily hurt to the native.

" Unfortunately, the man who flogged the native to death was not an uneducated outcast, but a member of a well-known English family, and a person of some status in society.

" Just as our ancestors objected to slavery, we now feel that something more must be done than leave the local natives to the local whites. The moral standard must be made effective wherever our jurisdiction goes. Where a small group of white men has power over a great number of natives, ordinary justice cannot be administered through the local opinion of a ruling class." Burns (C. D.), " Christian Nations and Others ", a Discourse, *The Monthly Record of South Place Ethical Society* (London, June, 1925), p. 6, a match was applied and the clothing burned from her person. When this had been done and while she was yet alive, a knife, evidently one such as used in splitting hogs, was taken and the woman's abdomen was cut open, the unborn babe falling from her womb to the ground. The infant, prematurely born, gave two feeble cries and then its head was crushed by a member of the mob with his heel."[1]

Paternal jealousy of the son certainly had an opportunity for expression in this last episode. That such events are but the too frequent accompaniment of the intolerence of the superior race, at least in the Land of Liberty, is borne out by the computation that

" During the last 30 years in the. United States 3,224 people—two or three every week—have been murdered by lynching mobs."[2]

" The vast majority have been perpetrated upon blacks by the whites whose culture they are alleged to menace, and often accompanied by a fiendishness never surpassed in Indian annals, eyes being gouged out by red hot pokers and slow fires built to prolong the victim's tortures."[3]

The incentive of a wish for father-like persecuting power seems clearly present in those who join, say, the Klu Klux Klan. At the same time, the secrecy of the order, and the regalia made of bleached vegetable fibre,[4] satisfy the opposed scruples. The activities of the organization, too, assist in this direction. It was primarily aimed to keep in subjection the negroes, whose sexual potency is so feared by the whites. Besides this, the Klan has taken under its special

---

[1] (Georgia, U.S.A., May, 1918). From Report of the National Annual Assoc. for Advancement of Coloured People, Jan., 1919. See also The Crisis, Sept., 1918 ; also pamphlet Lynching, May, 1918.

[2] Rowley (Dr Francis, H.), quoted in Haldeman Julius Monthly (Girard, Kan., March, 1925).

[3] Chicago Evening Post.

[4] In his lectures to the British Psycho-Analytical Association, in September, 1925, Dr Geza Roheim referred to instructions given to the ancient Egyptian priests, which at the earliest times said, not that they were to clothe themselves in white linen, but that they were to cover the penis therewith. Wool was forbidden the priests because it was hair and so symbolic of public parts and potency ; the priest shaved his entire body. Only with these symbols of castration might he enter the inner shrine (maternal womb),

protection the whole subject of the community morals. Thus in some cases it has punished women reputed to be promiscuous, by stripping and exposing them naked in the streets. This itself is of course a sexual gratification. All this is perhaps in part a neurotic reaction against inner guilt complexes, in part direct hatred of the son as rebel against the father, and in part cruelty to one's son as representing one's father[1] on the principle son = (his) grandfather. The conduct would be thus much over-determined, a fact which would help account for its ferocious strength.

All the foregoing discussion will help us to understand those humanitarian movements which are endeavouring to put down war, reform the prisons, abolish flogging and lynch-law, or help people to rise above racial snobbery as well as to mitigate cruelty to children and animals. Elements of genuine sympathy with suffering and of identification with the sufferer as a creature of our own kind, no doubt exist too in these movements. But besides being sometimes thus genuinely derived, humanitarianism must often be the fruit of reaction formations against echoes of ourselves of all these sinister motivations which impel to the brutal actions we have discussed.

In the present chapter we have seen how governments and the Klu Klux Klan persecuted rebel sons in fact, and Belloc in symbol, how the officials and old men and their following derived a satisfaction from military and penal institutions and from atrocities masking as measures to preserve our civilization, and how humanitarianism must often be a reaction-formation against such desires.

---

[1] Those familiar with Greek mythology will recall that in the revolt of the Titans against the gods, some few of the Titans sided with Zeus.

CHAPTER III

HOMOSEXUALITY, JEALOUSY FOR THE FATHER'S LOVE, AND IDENTIFICATION WITH HIM

INTRODUCTORY REMARKS

THE common conception of infancy as a period in which sex is yet indeterminate psychologically, is an overstatement, but not wholly a mis-statement, of the facts. While the young boy's love flows out chiefly to his mother, yet all who are reasonably kind to him normally receive their quota. This includes the father, even if toward him the son at the same time feels jealousy about his mother.

When his love towards his mother receives, for any reason, a check, the way is opened for a greater flood to be directed toward the father. Thus, Kenyon was very affectionate as a child towards his mother, whom he was ever wishing to fondle, and for whom he invented a variety of pet names. His mother had always manifested her love for him by championing him against his father, by studying his interests and making serious sacrifices on his behalf. Nevertheless, she early began to insist that his pet names for her were undignified, and to restrain excessive ardour in his childish demonstrations.[1]

---

[1] Among her own characteristics there seems to have been included a certain *malaise* in affective situations, which may well have resulted from the harsh discipline inflicted on her as a girl by her parents. For she had a tendency to ride rough-shod over people's feelings, especially when pursuing some benevolent end ; she admitted very few friends indeed to the intimacy of first names, and she retained a manner of greeting her children with a few kisses and an hour's conversation when they returned from across the continent or ocean, and then sending them about their business in such a way as to leave a doubt in their minds as to whether they were really wanted.

The son still remained fond of his mother, yet began to prefer two other persons to her. At the age of nine and a half he openly expressed a preference for his father. He also asked why the latter had not married a certain other woman who had acted as his foster-mother while the real parents were travelling. The libido thus directed to his father was in its turn eventually to receive a check, thus partly turning Kenyon back to his mother, but also contributing to a general affective sterility of any kind at all. Yet his temporary turning toward the father fixed in him permanently somewhat more than the average amount of homosexuality.

In the previous chapter I spoke of how, to the child, the father symbolizes power. But such power is by no means always inimical. Often it is exerted at the child's own behest. And so often as the father's strength, wisdom and authority are exerted for his son's defence or advancement, he becomes to the latter a rescuer, a source of refuge. In this capacity he has attributes in common with the hero, the saviour, the Christ. Generally, to be sure, these figures rather represent the child's super-ego, an ideal of what he himself would like to be, in rivalry of the father. Still, elements of father-admiration enter into the make-up of the *super-ego* itself.

I have mentioned having analysed a markedly homosexual neurotic whom I call Gould. He was the second of three brothers. His career of homosexual perversion in the physical sense commenced at the age of ten, when the youngest brother proposed pederasty to him, saying that the eldest brother had been practising it on him, the youngest. This eldest brother largely filled the rôle of the father, who had been for some time separated from his family. In doing as his eldest brother did, Gould was identifying himself with the absent father.

In the case cited in our introductory caption, just

above, the growing attachment of Kenyon to his father reacted upon him in a manner to make him then show some signs of jealousy against his mother, when the loved father gave her preference over Kenyon.

Such cases are not unusual. Freud remarks of jealousy

" that in many persons it is experienced bisexually ; that is to say, in a man, beside the suffering in regard to the loved woman and the hatred against the male rival, grief in regard to the unconsciously loved man and hatred of the woman as a rival will add to its intensity."[1]

The mechanism of *identification* is seen constantly in young children, who take up in play the activities of their parents. Upon the whole the tendency is to identify one's self chiefly with the parent of like sex ; and that this phenomenon is not absolutely dependent upon a positive transference is proven by Freud's example, somewhere in his *Collected Papers*, of a girl who bitterly hated her mother and yet mimicked the latter's mannerisms because she wished to be in her place in relation to her father. Yet, on the whole, identification seems to take place more readily when the subject is loved.

To the baby boy, his father is almost always a hero So long as the son retains a positive transference, this hero-worship is likely to endure, and to survive in a degree even the revelations which time is bound to effect, of the father's limitations. The father may die before this disillusionment takes place. In any case he is the first model after whom all future heroes must in however slight a degree, be copies ; and it was the child's adoration of him which fixed any part of the child's libido in the groove of hero-worship. Since king = father in the unconscious, father admiration may lead to king-worship.

The reverence which was originally paid the father

[1] Freud (S.), " Pathogenesis of a case of Homosexuality in a Woman ," in his *Collected Papers* (London, 1924), vol. II, p. 224.

is often transferred to God his surrogate, or to religion, or (as state worship) to the government.

Where the father is heroized, the qualities which characterized him will naturally come in for their measure of enhanced esteem.

Among these is likely to be, first of all, the attribute of power. That was generally the very earliest to call forth boyish admiration.

Following the age-old distinction which regards man as the volitional-intellectual and women as the emotional counterparts of each other, the boy will probably admire his father as a thinker. Wisdom and thought *per se* will thus receive added dignity ; whence an exaltation of science. On the other hand, the will may be selected for exaltation.

It is because that which we admire we in some measure strive to attain, that the loved father becomes the first model, after which the little son tries to form himself. A picture—perhaps taken from life simply, or perhaps improved upon—of the father, becomes the boy's first *super-ego*.

In some cases false ideals may be thus set up. The admiration for the power-commanding position of the father who has many employees, especially in his household, may lead through identification with him to a desire for, or illusion of actual need of, many servants.

As the father's love for his son may lead him to identify himself with the boy or his interests, so the reciprocal process also happens. Especially when the father is his boy's hero, the latter will show, by playing at his father's profession, wearing his father's hat, etc., sure signs of identification. Imitation is the outward sign, of which identification is generally the inward state.

Compared with his admired father, the son feels himself to be inferior. Relatively he is ignorant ; he aspires in imagination to the father's knowledge and intelligence.

We have a tendency to sympathize with those of whom we are fond. This is seen in very young children. William James somewhere mentions the case of a boy who sat intently watching his mother in a dentist's chair. Whenever she gave signs of pain, the child's face registered identical emotions. In the case of my own two-and-a-half-year-old son, I have observed distress and crying produced by his mother merely pretending to be hurt and to cry. The sympathizing person sees himself in the place of the other.

So in life at large, we tend to share the pleasures and unpleasures of others through identifying ourselves with them in imagination. And in this, the father-minded are not so alienated from those whom they regard in the light of sons, but what feelings of sympathy may break through or at times (though not always) even overcome the more hostile feelings already described, e.g. the older generation may feel pity for the young men while it is sending them to the battlefield.

ECONOMICO-POLITICAL TYPE OF MOVEMENTS

The son who feels himself to be united closely and without clash with the father, cannot easily understand those who speak of an opposition of interests. Witness how conservatives generally construe the Marxian doctrine that war necessarily exists between the owning class and the working class, as being a preachment that such a war should be begun. An anti-socialist book similarly denies the viewpoint we noted on page 29, in as dogmatic terms as those in which Lenin asserted it :

> " Division of society into two classes—those who possess the implements of production and those who do not—is arbitrary and absurd."[1]

[1] *Anti-Socialist Union Speakers' Handbook* (London, 1911), p. 113.

While generally allying himself with the sons, Karl Marx seems yet in many respects to have felt himself to be of the fathers. I have already mentioned the episode of his breaking relations with his disciple Hyndman when this faithful son put on Marx's (phallically symbollic) headpiece. We have seen, moreover, that Màrx possessed the " God-complex " with its involved tendency to identify oneself with the (heavenly) father.[1] On the other hand, in the conservative camp we find " X·——" going beyond the point of ordinary loyalty and appearing quite to identify himself with the father, through whose eyes he views all political problems :

> " These addresses have a common theme . . . the fundamental principles [of] American Government and American civil society. . . . The Fathers would have been amazed at the notion that within a century and a half there would arise in America those who would . . . deny . . . the underlying moral and political principles upon which America is based."[2]

" X——'s " advice to us all is, that we become one with the fathers by steeping ourselves in their wisdom, and making their holy utterances our own, so we shall speak, as it were, with their voice :

> " Every American . . . should learn by heart the preamble to the Constitution of the United States. He should also . . . study the *Federalist*, which is the very Bible of our American form of government. He should know accurately the contents of Washington's Farewell

---

[1] A father-resembling aspect of the God-complex in Marx was his abnormal secretiveness :—
" One of his chief confidents was Eccarius, a Greek tailor, whom, however, he never seems to have trusted completely. That, all through, was his weakness ; he was intimate also with the English Trade Union leaders, Applegarth, Odger and Allen ; all were men of intelligence and character, but in none of them did he repose perfect confidence. At the same time he liked to have someone on whom he could rely and to whom he could go for advice if required." Salter (F. R.), *Karl Marx and Modern Socialism* (London, 1921), p. 45.
[2] " X——," *Is A. W. S. ?* (London, 1920), Introduction, p. ix.

Address, and he should be able to recite from memory Lincoln's Address at Gettysburg, and his Second Inaugural."[1]

RELIGIO-THERAPEUTIC TYPE

Nearly all religions have some sacrament representing union or reunion with the father, which sacrament we significantly call *communion*. Generally this consists in a ceremonial eating of his flesh (reunion by incorporation after slaying). The American Red Indians seem to have looked on their smoking ceremonial as a means of reunion through ecstacy.

Now, William James contends that :

> " In . . . the religious ecstacies it is difficult to exclude the possibility of an important part being played by the idea of an external person, namely, God. This is, of course, more evident in the trances of Christian saints than in those of other mystics ; but it is worthy of note that even in the Indian form of mysticism the word yoga is defined as ' the experimental union of the individual with the divine '."[2]

So far as the father is a loved figure, he will almost certainly impersonate for the son the qualities of goodness and goodwill. This is partly owing to idealization on the part of the son, and partly because the actual possession of these traits by the father is one of those factors which will have predisposed the son to love him as a father-substitute.

The desired union with the father may be striven after through dances and exercises, or it may be treated by the unconscious as existing, as where one identifies oneself with God.

---

[1] " X——," *Is A. W S.?* (London, 1920), p. x.
[2] James (Wm.), *Varieties of Religious Experiences*, 1902, p. 400.

Sacred Dancing and Exercises

In ancient Egypt,

" In the first dynasty the crown prince danced before the king at the installation festival . . . "[1]

Games, exercises and dances in honour of a deity, were, of course, common among the ancient Greeks,[2] the Therapeutæ and the Essenes,[3] and derivatively from the Therapeutæ, the modern Sufis.[4]

[1] " At later occasions the king danced various ritual dances, which are figured on the monuments. Dancing was a feature of the Bubastis festival. At funerals there was a dance circling round, which may be seen continued at present ; one woman will stand beating a tambourine, and half-a-dozen others will circle round her, shrieking and wailing. This will be repeated at every hundred yards on the way to the cemetery.

" The dances represented on the tombs of the old kingdom seem to be mostly performances for show, such as the high kick ; but these performed with wands, by a company all kicking in unison, may well have been in a regular ritual." Petrie (Prof. Sir F.), in a lecture at University College, November 8th, 1923.

[2] " Festivals called ' Hermaia ' seem to have been fairly common in Greece. . . . From a few references in *Pinder* it would appear that the Hermais at Pollene in Achaia was the most celebrated ; it was also called the Oeogevia, as if Hermes were the host of the other deities on this occasion. We hear only of athletic contests on these occasions ; there is no record of artistic or musical competitions." Farnell (L. B.), *Cults of the Greek States*, v. 5, p. 32.

[3] " The Therapeutæ confined themselves to a life of contemplation ; they were a small community of men and women who had been well born and wealthy and who lived in a Chartreuse-like retreat ; they were not religious communists and they had no interest in prophecy (their dreams being not of the future, but of the celestial order), they fasted, as the Essenes did not, and their relation to women was quite different. Both the Therapeutæ and the Essenes were ' holiness ' movements, but the former displayed some unique features, especially the combination of individual contemplation with an outburst of emotional fervour in the common song and dance." Summarization from Philo : *De Vita Contemplativa*, by Moffatt (J.), in art. " Therapeutæ ", in *Encyclopædia of Religion and Ethics*.

" Once every seven weeks they assemble for their supreme festival ' which the number fifty has had assigned to it ', robed in white and with looks of serious joy. At a given sign from one of their leaders, they arrange themselves in ranks, raising eyes and hands to heaven (' their hands because they are pure from unjust gains, being stained by no pretence of money making '), and praying for a blessing on the festival. Then the senior members recline, in order of seniority, upon their cheap rough couches, on the left side of the room the women also recline. The younger novices wait upon the elder members.

[4] Thus Professor Flinders Petrie says : " The æsthetic Therapeutæ in the first century A.D. greatly used dancing. At their great gathering, held every seven weeks, they ' keep the holy all-night festival . . . one

Indeed—and this point is important—the very name, Dhikr, which these last give to their ecstatic exercises of the type of the one I have described at length a few pages back, seems to indicate that they are intended essentially as expressions of loyalty to the Heavenly Father :

> " Dhikr in the mind (bilkalb) means ' Remembrance ', and with the tongue (Bil-lisan) ' mentioning ', ' relating ' then, as a religious technical term (pronounced zikr) the glorifying of Allah . . . with peculiar breathings and physical movements and . . . the repetition a great number of times of such phrases as la ilaha illa 'llah, subhana 'llah, al hamdu billah, allahu akbar, astarghfiru 'llah and the different names of Allah. Spiritual songs, often indistinguishable from love songs, may be introduced, as also dancing "[1]

Among the sects of Dervishes practising the Dhikr may be mentioned the Sa'dites,[2] the Baiyumiya,[3] and others, some of which will be considered under other heads below.

This motive is well recognized as important in all the

hand beating time to the answering chant of the other ' like a modern zikr of country folk ; ' dancing to its music . . . turning and returning in the dance '." Petrie (Prof. Sir Flinders), Lecture at University College, November 8th, 1923.
Macdonald tells that " This practice is based ultimately on Kuran, xxxiii, 41. ' O ye who believe, remember (or glorify) Allah with much remembering (or glorifying)'. A tradition from Muhammad is also frequently quoted : ' There sits not a company remembering (or glorifying) Allah, but the angels surround and the (Divine) mercy covers them, and Allah Most High remembers (or glorifies) them among those who are with him.' " Macdonald (D. B.), in art. " Dhikr ", in Encyclopædia of Islam.

[1] The passage continues : " At the regular Friday service (had ra) in the takiya or zawiya, which all dervishes are expected to attend the ritual consists especially in the formula La illaha illa 'llah, called the hzib or ' office ' in the technical sense of the order, which is made up of extended selections from the Koran and other prayers." Macdonald (D. B.), in art. " Dhikr ", in Encyclopædia of Islam.

[2] " The Sa'dites used to have the Dawsa and still in their monasteries use the beating of little drums, called Baz. The use of these is now forbidden in the Egyptian mosques, as an innovation (bida : Muhammad Abduh, Tarikh, II, 44 et seq." Macdonald (D. B.), art. " Dervishes ", in Encyclopædia of Islam.

[3] " Its founder . . . renewed the ritual of the Badawiya, to which he gave a more stimulating character and made stricter by more stringent exercises. . . . The dhikr of the order consists in calling out ya Allah ! with an inclination of the head and crossing of the hands on the breast, followed by raising the head and clapping the hands." Huart (C,), in art. " Baiyumia ", in Encyclopædia of Islam,

sthenic sects to which allusion has been made—this wish for union with the (heavenly) father. In its broader sense, probably none of them would deny this. A repressed element therein is found, however, in the sensuous nature which this longing manifests. In dreams[1] rhythmic motion commonly symbolizes coitus, whether normal or perverted ; and the connection is often equally to the fore in religious festivals, as among the ancient Greeks,[2] the Hebrews,[3] the Tantricas, of course, and the Therapeutæ.[4]

[1] My (markedly homosexual) analysand, Gould, once brought me the following account of a dream : " The changes of duration and position produce, by virtue of the persistence of impulse, a melody of sensations. This dance is, at times, slow and snake-like in its sequence ; at others like the battle roar of a gun. At times it produces a tantalising rhythm—the suspense and change between long and short duration drives one almost mad. At times a graceful impulse starts ascending, then changes to some horizontal form. When I have become oriented to this horizontal impulse, it changes to some parabolic form. It makes one feel like cubic art. However, when the dance was finished, I felt no broken impulse-strands. I felt all impulses had been a part of one great unity."

[2] Speaking of the rites of Artemis, Farnell observes : " There is another feature occasionally discernable in her worship, namely, orgiastic and lascivious dances and the use of phallic emblems in the ritual. At Ellis . . . we hear of . . . the worship being accompanied with the dance that Pausanias considers to be native to the region of Sipylos and to have been brought into the Elean cult by the followers of Pelops ; and at Derrha on Taygetus, where Artemis was worshipped, we hear of a dance of the same character . . . performed in her honour." Farnell, *Cults of the Greek States*, vol. 2, p. 445.

[3] " The root which is the one most frequently used in the Old Testament for dancing, viz. *hul* . . . expresses the ' whirl ' of the dance (e.g. Judg. xxi, 21, 23 ; Ps. I, xxxvii, 7). It is the word used in the sense of dancing, contortions of the body are thought of, which suggest something of a rather wild character." Oesterley (W. O. E.), *The Sacred Dance*, 1923, p. 45.

[4] " For their supreme festival. . . . The final act of the festival is the famous . . . all night celebration of a sacred singing dance, by men and women in two choruses each headed by a chosen leader. Each of the choirs, the male and the female, begins by singing and dancing apart, partly in unison, partly in antiphonal measures of various metres, ' as if it were a Bacchic festival in which they had drunk deep of the divine love '.

" Then both unite to imitate the choral (Ex. 15, 1, 20-1) songs of Moses and Miriam at the Red Sea, sung as thanks, cf. Rev. 15. It is a thrilling performance, this Choric dance, and exulting symphony, ' but the end and aim of all is holiness ' (the exodus symbolising, of course, the mystical release of the soul from material bondage)." Philo, *De Vita Contemplativa*, as quoted by Moffatt (F.), in art. " Therapeutæ ", in *Encyclopædia of Religion and Ethics*,

Of the performances of the Dervishes at Kairoan, which I have described, the sexual significance was evident. The rhythmic nature of the chanting and swaying, the ecstatic state induced, the slow attainment of each individual of a climax, and the unmistakably sensual expression of some of the dancers, all pointed to this conclusion.

The use of the dance to induce sensuous states is practised by the sects described, and by the Mawlawites[1] and others. In all the Sufi fraternities some closely analogous form of ritual is followed,[2] in which the largely homosexual love motive is indicated by the presence in some degree of the symptoms above mentioned. Where there is not actual dancing, there is apt at least to be some rhythmic swaying in time to a chant. Macdonald gives the following description of a ceremony he witnessed :

" They began to recite, rapidly and in cadence, certain religious formulæ. . . . They accompanied these, however, with certain motions and gestures of the head and body, and by great care, evidently, with regard to breathing.

" For example, one of the most frequent recurring elements was the Muslim confession of faith, *La ilaha illa llah,* ' There is no God save Allah ', and it had evidently to be performed in a certain way. At *La ilaha,* ' There is no God ', the head of each went down in front of one shoulder ; this is the phrase of denial ; the nothingness of all things is to be felt. Then at *illa-llah* ' except Allah ', the head went down in front of the other shoulder. This second phrase is assertion, and the absoluteness of Allah's existence must be felt. This movement also directed and controlled the breathing. The

---

[1] " The Mawlawites, founded by Djalal al-Din Al-Rumi (d. at Konia in 672 A.H.) stimulate their ecstasies by a whirling dance." Macdonald (D. B.), in art. " Dervishes ", in *Encyclopædia of Islam.*

[2] " The religious service common to all fraternities is called a *Dikr,* a ' remembering ' that is, of Allah (Kur xxxiii, 41 is the basal text), and its object is to bring home to the worshipper the thought of the unseen world and of his dependence upon it. Further, it is plain that a *Dikr* brings with it a certain heightened religious exaltation and a pleasant dreaminess. But there go also with the hypnosis, either as excitants or consequents, certain physical states and phenomena which have earned for Dervishes the various descriptions in the West of barking, howling, dancing, etc." Macdonald (B. D.), in art, " Der-vishes ", in *Encyclopædia of Islam.*

recitation and movement gradually grew faster and faster, heads going from side to side in perfect time, head down at the one point, down at the other. . . .
" If the breathing is regulated in a certain way in the utterance of such formulæ as these, the emotional effect is increased."[1]

The participant in these ceremonies may then rationalize his motives, making it appear that these aimed at sthenic or other benefits experienced as the result of the exercises.[2]

If we now examine a modern cult, Mazdaznan, which has yet more recently begun to flourish in America, we shall find features in it similar to some among the Sufis. This cult obviously comes within the meaning of the terms sthenic and therapeutic, for it advertises itself as a system of self-development, gains its adherents through a correspondence course in which they are taught homely facts about the care of their bodies and minds, and includes in its ritual the performance of physical exercises. Among other things, the adherent is bidden to :

" Kneel at the back of a chair, bending both knees at the same time. . . . After the prelude breaths, inhale fully and deeply, at the same time tightening the grasp. . . .
" There will be nothing you cannot grasp and understand, and then you will comprehend that even the light which you thought comes from the sun is but the light of our own planet . . . that our planet is a light unto itself, and that ' I am the Light of the World '.
" Remaining in the position described, with all ideas

---

[1] Macdonald (D. B.), *Aspects of Islam*, 1911, pp. 160-4.
[2] Macdonald says : " It was perfectly evident that the young men who were taking part were intensely interested in it all. . . . It was certainly a thing into which they threw themselves with zest. . . . I think they got out of it at first a certain heightening of religious emotion . . . and . . . a certain effect of auto-hypnosis. They produced in themselves a pleasant dreaminess. The attraction evidently lay in a very curious mixture of æsthetic pleasures—derived from the nerve tension and the highly hypnotic, or hypnoidal, state into which they were cast—and undoubtedly religious exaltation. The latter element was certainly there. . . .
" I wish to say as emphatically as possible that I did feel . . . that behind all this there was a real devotional spirit." Macdonald (D. B.), *Aspects of Islam*, 1911, pp. 163-5.

banished from your mind, follow the current of inhalation as it enters the nostrils, the air tubes and the lungs ; forget even the names of Ga Llama, the centralizing life principle, even Breathing, in fact. . . . For the first time you will feel an inner charming power that will captivate you, and, repeating this exercise, a burning will be felt, yet so soothing, so pacifying, that it will seem like the unfoldment of some fairyland.   And again through repetition a wonderful light will appear—the light of the soul.   It will illustrate your mind, warm your heart, set into ecstacy, as it were, your physical functions.   Then draw all your thoughts from the circumference around you into your inmost self, and a sweet, soft breeze as the blowing of the north wind will linger around you, scattering delicious fragrance like the perfume of roses.   You will feel a degree of grandeur no tongue or language will be able to express.   Still on and on you will continue to go on this plane of eternal progression to which there is no end."[1]

Apparently what happens here is, that the Mazdaznan devotee first places himself in the conventional posture of homage to the heavenly father.   The heightened oxidation and rhythmic action of the breathing exercise then aids him to induce in himself the ecstatic condition which most mystics describe as a sense of union with the father.   The above passage emphasizes the ecstatic element in this cult ; the one below brings out most forcibly the attitude of father-adoration.

" Exercise six.
" We now come to an exercise where all people bow their knees.   There is a time in every mans' life, whether Jew or Gentile, heathen or Christian, when he should bow his knee in reverence.   The principle object of this exercise is to distribute the magnetic circles for aiding in the awakening of the spinal cord, thus expanding the realms of thought, enabling you to reason more logically and be able to perceive through the sense of feeling the inner physical mechanism of your being, guiding you by virtue of the activity of the brain cells to the unfoldment of a perfect consciousness and realization that you are one with God and nature."[2]

[1] Ha'nish (O. Z.), *Mazdaznan Health and Breath Culture*, pp. 121-2.
[2] *Idem*, p. 121.

In Rome at Eastertime, and at the cathedral in Valencia (I believe at Christmas) and a few other places, a special choir of boys still performs a dance in honour of the heavenly father. But in general this custom is less usual in christendom than beyond its borders.

Let us now consider a nonconformist sect who, in imitation of Jesus, lay great stress on healing the sick, namely the Seventh Day Adventists. Very retrograde in their theology, but yet progressive in their therapy, they feel forced to condemn social dancing as a sinful pastime displeasing to the heavenly father, while yet they recognize the physiological and psychological value of rhythmic exercises socially enjoyed. Their solution of the problem thus raised is an ingenious one. At their enormous Sanitarium at Battle Creek, Michigan, which was of Adventist origin, and its numerous branches, the patients are gathered together in the gymnasium, which is always a large hall. All the young and robust members, together with men and women nurses and doctors, then line up for *marching*. They go through a great variety of steps, and of exercises of all sorts, to music. It is a sort of choral performance, and greatly enjoyed. It is significant that the more cynical patients name this marching " sterilized dancing ".

Self-identification with God

We have seen how Christ, regarded as " one with the father ", is so even when the father meant is the earthly one. It follows that a desire to be Christ-like may often conceal a wish to be father-like. Moxon tells us :

" When infantile self-love is overlaid by the higher state of object love, the child identifies itself with the beloved parent who is loved like a god. By this introjection of the parent into the self, the child can offer a willing obedience. To obey the parent is to obey one's self. This psychical stage in religion is represented by the joy and freedom felt by the child of God in a slavish service to his will."[1]

When the father who is most revered is at a remove of several generations, identification of self with him may be facilitated, and the power of his authority passes down more easily, when the whole sequence from ancestral figures to the present generation is known most clearly and in most detail. This contention is born out by the emphasis which has always been put on direct and legitimate descent. We see it operative in the Sufi religion, where each Dervish makes a great point of the Silsila or "chain" by which he is connected through the *imaum* who taught him, and so on back to Mohammed, to the angel Gabriel, who brought revelation to Mohammed, and finally to Allah.[2]

This seems to represent the passing on of the seed (impregnation by the father). The prophet, of course, is a surrogate for God—in so considering him, his followers do but regard him as he usually, whether unwittingly or not, regards himself.[3]

We have seen how Quimby equated *wisdom* with the father. We shall now find him speaking of his therapy

[1] " In the boy there soon arise the iconoclastic forces of jealousy in regard to the mother and rebellious hatred of paternal authority. Consequently the father is now felt to be an inadequate ideal and the boy may take as father-substitute some real or imaginary hero who for a time can satisfy the emotional needs. With adolescence, however, comes the increased critical power to see that even heroes have feet of clay. If the Oedipus complex is still dominant, new sublimations are now required, such as patriotic love of the Fatherland, or religious love of the Father God." Moxon (C.), " A Psycho-analytical study of the Christian Creed ", *The International Journal of Psycho-Analysis* (London, 1921), vol. II.

[2] Macdonald (D. B.), in art. " Dervishes ", in *Encyclopædia of Islam.*

[3] " To the common people the figures of Buddha, Mahomet, Peter and Moses mean something more than mere representatives of God, and we find even minor prophets and preachers speaking in the name of God with an authority so astounding as to preclude the idea of its arising solely in learning ; in other words, one feels sure that their conscious attitude is generally the product of an unconscious phantasy in which they identify their personality with God." Jones (E.), " The God Complex ", published in the *Internationale Zeitschrift fur Psychoanalyse*, 1913, Bd. I, S. 313. Republished in his *Essays in Applied Psycho-Analysis* (London, 1923), p, 205.

as so guided by his father that we must consider that he thought of father, wisdom and self as identical :

"My practice is not of the wisdom of man. . . . Jesus said, 'If I judge of myself, my opinion is not good, but if I judge of God, it is right '. . . . So if I judge as a man it is an opinion, and you can get plenty of them anywhere. . . . "My practice . . . belongs to a Wisdom that is above man as man."[1]

Quimby also admits others to this privilege of identity with the father. The sentence in which he tells us so may well banish any remaining doubt of the equation, wisdom—father.

"Every man is a part of God just so far as he is wisdom."[2]

If in the case of Quimby we must rest content with indirect inferences of an identification which was *not openly* avowed, such is not the case with his pupil. There can be no mistaking the announcement in the *Christian Science Journal* that :

"Mrs Eddy has distinctly authorized the claims on her behalf that she herself was . . . the chosen successor to, and equal of, Jesus."[3]

The president of the Christian Science Congress in the following year was permitted to give out the following confirmation of these divine pretensions :

"There is one Moses, one Jesus, and one Mary."[4]

Marden, the New Thought writer, in his *Every Man a King*, in a chapter significantly entitled "The Coming Man Will Realize His Divinity ", quotes on how we come into

"One-ness with the blessed One. . . . He who sees God in All feels the ecstatic and blissful thrill of the Infinite

---

[1] Quimby (P. P.), "Letter to a Clergyman ", October 28th, 1860. Quoted by Dresser (A.G.), *Philosophy of P. P. Quimby* (Boston, 1895), p. 54.
[2] Quimby (P.P.), see Dresser (H. W.), *Quimby Manuscripts* (New York), p. 408.
[3] *Christian Science Journal*, April, 1899. Quoted by Wirgman (The Ven. Archdeacon), (Port Elizabeth, 1917).
[4] President of Christian Science Congress, in 1890, in message to Mrs Eddy. Quoted by Wirgman.

Presence that cannot be described. How beautiful is the Universe to Him who is one with the Planner and knows the Plan."[1]

We have thus far had to do almost wholly with God as the father-substitute through whom identification is traced. Other surrogates, however, occur; and an especially frequent type is some older person whom a young man reads about or meets, and who becomes his hero. Such a mechanism seems to have played a chief part in determining the career of Emile Coué.

" It was in 1885, at the age of twenty-eight, that M. Coué met Liébault, and without any doubt this meeting decided the course of his life. Liébault was . . . a country doctor, unambitious and unpretentious . . . Coué's career was of a somewhat similar type. He has always shown the same modesty; he never goes to see people, but waits for them to come to him, he has never pushed himself forward.

" Having witnessed Liébault's experiments, he started himself to practise suggestion."[2]

Here Liébault, clearly, was a father-figure for Coué.

This is all I have to say on the subject of identification. In this chapter of our thesis we have seen how identification with the father led to reverence for his voice in politics, and in religion to dances and to gestures and expressions of union and hero-worship.

---

[1] Quoted from " The Blissful Prophet ", by Marden (O. S.), *Every Man a King* (London), chap. xxi, p. 231.
[2] Lady Noble of Ardinglas: *Coué and Auto-Suggestion.*

CHAPTER IV

PROVIDENCE

Introductory Remarks

IT is the experience of the very young babe, that everything is done for him. He has but to utter a cry, and someone comes running to minister to his wants. Unwise parents continue this regime too long into childhood. They make their young hopeful dependent upon their efforts instead of upon his own.

In the often mentioned instance of Kenyon, this was the case. The father had amassed for him a fortune which relieved him for all time of any necessity for earning his living. One of his early memories was that of standing on the deck of a ship in the Bay of Naples, and shuddering as he gazed down on a group of raggamuffins scuffling upon the wharf. " But for my father's wealth ", he thought, " I should have to fight for my place among rough boys like these ! "[1]

[1] It is uncertain, however, how much a tremendous inferiority-complex and its concomitant tendency to rely upon others, which Kenyon exhibited, were due to his father ; for it seems due at least as much to his mother. The latter had an executive managerial *flair*, which had been developed by the fact that her husband, as an invalid, came to leave an increasing number of responsibilities to his wife's care. She took a far more active part in arranging her son's life than was wise ; as an observer once said, she still " brooded over " him like a hen over her lone chick, when he was a man past thirty ! (Indeed, " chick " is a pet name she still gives him at forty). She was wont to say (rationalization) that in her own childhood she had been made to take so many responsibilities, that she swore that if ever she had a child of her own, he should have no responsibilities at all ! Those familiar with Russian literature will recall the fiction-character of Oblomoff, who was enfeebled by similar means. Freud (S.), " The Economic Problem in Masochism ", first published in *Zeitschrift*, Bd. X, 1924. (Translated by Joan Riviere). Published in *Collected Papers* (London, 1924), vol. II, p. 265.

The father, moreover, was a chronic invalid who exploited his invalidism as a means of shirking responsibilities. This, through the working of the identification-complex of which we shall presently speak, worked with other influences to make Kenyon likewise irresponsible.

The boy early rejected all theological beliefs. But in this his case was unusual under the circumstances. Images of the earthly parents in most such cases become exalted into the conception of Heavenly Father and of mother-nature respectively. One may generally count on childish experiences of the benevolent foresight of father or mother becoming sublimated into a trust in Providence or in the kindly wisdom of nature. But Kenyon's father himself was a sceptic.

The attributes ascribed to God are generally an index of infantile experiences of the earthly father. The God of a patriarchal people is himself an arbitrary, stern deity, commanding them to butcher their enemies, sack cities, and sell whole populations into slavery. As the ethics of a people improve, those of the deity at length follow suit.

At an advanced stage of culture, three ideas especially —namely, those of paternal power, wisdom and goodness—are abstracted from the weaknesses and mortality of the earthly father, and made attributes of his heavenly prototype. We then call God the All-loving One, All-animating One (= the Fertilizer or Creator), the benevolent Thinker, Providence, etc. His manifestation, Nature, is endowed with purpose.

But, warns Freud,

> " All those who transfer the guidance of the world to Providence, to God, or to God and Nature, rouse a suspicion that they still look upon these farthest and remotest powers as a parent-couple—mythologically—and imagine themselves linked to them by libidinal bonds."[1]

[1] Freud (S.), " The Economic Problems in Masochism ", first published in *Zeitschrift*, Bd. X, 1924. (Translated by Joan Riviere). Published in *Collected Papers* (London, 1924), vol. II, p. 265.

Flügel, likewise, comments upon

" the unwillingness of men to abandon a certain childlike attitude in virtue of which they are prone to believe that all their needs will in some manner be provided for without the necessity for forethought or effort on their own part. . . .
    " It finds expression in such well-known phrases as ' Bountiful Nature ', and ' Providence never sends mouths but it sends food '."[1]

The mode of working this complex may be illustrated from the case of a writer who recalls, as a boy,

" taking many foolish and dangerous risks in climbing and on the river, which I should not have ventured to do, but for the firm belief that God had already determined the day of my death and that nothing I could do would alter it."[2]

[1] " (Statements which every serious student of biology and economics knows to be profoundly untrue in the sense that is intended) and may be regarded as a particular aspect of a more general view, according to which the care of men is entrusted to the hands of a beneficent and ever watchful deity, whose constant vigilance relieves the human race of the necessity for foresight and makes it a virtue to ' take no thought for the morrow ' since to do otherwise would imply distrust of, or disbelief in, the deity in question. In the light of psycho-analysis it is easy to see that this attitude is principally derived (1) from the positive (or loving) elements of the parent regarding complexes, the unlimited power and beneficence originally attributed to the parents being displaced on to the more abstract personalities of God or Nature ; (2) from displaced Narcissistic tendencies." Flügel (J. C.), " Biological basis of Sexual Repression ", *British Journal of Medical Psychology*, 1925, vol. I.

[2] " My position was quite logical. I was told that God knew everything, without any limitation whatever. He not only knew everything that had happened, everything that was now happening, but he knew everything that was going to happen in the future. Therefore, it naturally followed that he knew the day of my death ; it was settled and unalterable by anything I could do. I have no doubt that many accidents to life and limb are due to this superstition.
    " It is a belief much more widely spread than most people imagine, and among all ranks of society. In reading the reminiscences of Prof. the Rev. A. H. Sayce, the orientalist, we come across the following confession :—
    " ' There was one conviction, however, which was more deeply rooted than any other, and is still as strong as it was in the dawn of my life. I knew, as I knew nothing else, that everything is determined beforehand, and that whatever happens—at all events to oneself— is in accordance with the decree of an inexorable and passionless fate. The conviction has stood me in good stead in my later years ; I have never hesitated about carrying out a plan for fear of the personal consequences ; when what the orient terms " the day " arrives, we must die, whatever we may be doing or wherever we may be ; before that day arrives we are destined to live '." *The Freethinker* (London, 1925).

The ancient Essenes, so we are told by Philo, regarded "the Deity as the cause of all good and no evil, thus forestalling, among others, the Christian Science and New Thought writers whom we shall presently mention.

In the New Testament, of course, an expression of the trust in Providence as being better than personal effort is to be found in the admonition to be guided by the example of the lilies of the field which do not toil nor spin, and by the birds of the air over whom the Heavenly Father watches.

So opposite a thinker from Jesus as was Karl Marx had yet in him a vein of providential trust, in that he was assured of the ultimate triumph of his ideas

> " because he thought that they proceeded along the lines pre-ordained by the nature of things."[1]

Economico-Political Type of Movement

The dilution of sound economic theory by the notion that Providence will somehow make everything come all right, is most apparent where distinctly religious ideas are intermingled in the argument.

> "Where did the false idea of . . . the necessity of competition, originate?' It had its origin in the pessimistic assumption that it is impossible for everyone to be wealthy or successful; in the thought of limitation of all things which most men desire; and that, there not being enough for all . . . the shrewdest . . . will get the most of it.

---

[1] Marx, who had within him a strong vein of contra·iety and pugnacity, says in another place, in reply to some disparagement of Hegel: 'I therefore announced myself the pupil of that mighty thinker, and then and there in the chapter on the theory of value, coquetted with the modes of expression peculiar to him.'

"One notion which he derived from Hegel gave him a certain spirit of faith, though it does not add to the value of his analysis of economic conditions. This might be expressed as the principle of Determinism.

"Marx became assured of the ultimate triumph of his ideas because he thought that they proceeded along the lines pre-ordained by the nature of things." *Freethinker* (London, November 30th, 1924).

This theory is fatal to all individual and race betterment."
[i.e. it shall be untrue, because it would deny our wishes.]
" The Creator never put vast multitudes of people on
this earth to scramble for a limited supply, as though he were
not able to furnish enough for all. There is nothing in the
world which men desire and struggle for, and that is good
for them, of which there is not enough for everybody."[1]

Again, the same writer, with an implication that
he is initiated into the secrets of the father, tells us :

" We were made . . . to be prosperous. The trouble
with us is that we do not trust the law of infinite supply,
but close our natures so that abundance cannot flow to
us. . . .
" Our pinched, dwarfed, blighted lives come from in-
ability to be united with the great Source of all supply."[2]
(Desire for union with the father).

Thus the world's alleged problems are no problems
at all ; economics and sociology are foolishness. For
if we are but good trustful children, father will bring us
whatever we want.

" When man comes into the full realization that God is
his never failing Supply, the Source of abundance, the great
Fountain Head of all that is good and desirable, and that
he being His offspring must be part, an indestructible part,
of this Supply, he will never more know poverty nor lack
of any kind."[3]

Mrs Hyndman, in her biography of H. M. Hyndman,
attributed to him great optimism of temperament.
This, she said, made him somewhat blind to those
"dark Asian strands " in human nature, which might
provide further obstacles to the quick realization of
universal happiness in place of those which socialism
removed. Apparently Hyndman regarded Marx as
Providence, whose word, *Das Kapital*, was sufficient
to straighten all things for his children.

In order to account for the success with which a

[1] Marden (O. S.), *Peace, Power and Plenty* (London, 1909), pp. 38-9.
[2] *Idem*, pp. 41, 44.
[3] *Idem*, p. 49.

certain movement has met, it is sometimes said to have appeared upon the scene at the moment when the stage was especially prepared by God, fate, or chance, i.e. providentially :

> " In order that the socialism of the present day might assume so quickly that religious form which constitutes the secret of its power, it was necessary that it should appear at one of these rare moments in history when the old religions lose their might (men being weary of their Gods) and exist only on sufferance, while awaiting the new faith that is to succeed them. Socialism coming as it came at the precise instant when the power of the old divinities had considerably waned, is naturally tending to possess itself of their place."[1]

Protectionism owes rather less to the motive we are now considering than do most movements. For, if you trust in Providence, there is nothing to protect against. Under the rule of Providence all things must be for the best. But, therefore, the providentially-minded person cannot believe that anything—least of all his own favourite movement—may owe its success to being pushed by an influential interested minority and not to it being for the general good :

> " Protection never could have made headway if it had operated to make things actually and permanently dearer."[2]

All ultra-rational faith in any movement has in it presumably a certain providential element.

Politically, the faith in Providence, or the father's all-comprehensive vigilance, is apt to be shown in an easy-going confidence that our rulers will do what is right, and that it is unnecessary for each of us individually to take an active part in practical politics.

This spirit better suits autocratic than democratic institutions. So soon as the citizen feels that his civic duty is summarized in the pithy admonition of a U.S.

---

[1] Le Bon (G.), *Psychology of Socialism* (London), p. 12.
[2] Young (J. P.), *Protection and Progress* (Chicago and New York, 1900), p. 11.

attorney-general in 1918, " Obey the law, and keep
your mouth shut ", i.e. be like a good child, seen but
not heard, so soon are all defences against arbitrary
government let down.

In times of distress, the providentially-minded tend
to look for help, not to themselves, but to some father-
surrogate.   I have mentioned how in that very religious
country, India, a few years ago, I was much impressed
by the frequency with which I heard the refrain, " Let
government (father) do it ! "   So also, as a writer in
Psyche, last year, truthfully observed :

> " The demand for the strong man, the Mussolini, [is]
> unconsciously the babe's cry for daddy and mother to kiss
> the sore place and make it well again."[1]

Humanitarian Type of Movement

Exalted faith in the providential arrangement of
the world and the rational (fatherlike) nature of mankind shone through the prophecy of I. S. Block in 1890
that

> " there will be no war in the future, for it has become
> impossible now that it is clear that war means suicide."[2]

The same may be said of a like prediction by David
Starr Jordan as late as 1913.   His childlike trust in the
banker-fathers, etc., was touching :

> " What shall we say of the Great War of Europe ever
> threatening, ever impending, and which never comes ?   We
> shall say that it will never come. Humanly speaking, it
> is impossible. . . . The bankers will not find the money
> for such a fight, the industries of Europe will not maintain
> it, the Statesmen cannot. . . . The Masters have much to

---

[1] *Psyche* (London, May, 1924). (?).
[2] Block (I. S.), *Future of War*, 1899. Quoted by Maxim (Hudson),
Defenceless America (London, New York, Toronto), p. 1.

gain, but vastly more to lose, and their signal will not be given."[1]

But it is by no means only pacifists who have found support in this view that father arranges all things for the best. Some have seen in war itself the Father to whom we owe our very being, and the Divine Author of all the good in the world. (The harshness and discipline of war suit it to a father rôle.) In the ranks of these worshipful sons, we are surprised to find Ruskin :

" War . . . is the foundation of all the high virtues and faculties of men. . . . The common notion that peace and the virtues of civil life flourish together I have found to be utterly untenable. Peace and the vices of civil life only flourish together. We talk of peace and learning, of peace and plenty, of peace and civilization ; but I found that these are not the words that the Muse of History couples together. That on her lips the words were peace and sensuality, peace and selfishness, peace and death. I found in brief that all great nations learned their truth of word and strength of thought in war ; That they were nourished in war and wasted in peace ; taught by war and deceived by peace . . . born in war and expired in peace."
" All the pure and noble arts of peace are founded on war ; no great art ever arose on earth but among a nation of soldiers. There is no great art possible to a nation but that which is based on battle."[2]

The eulogies of war by Nietzsche, Treitschke, etc. (based largely upon a distorted version of the Darwinian hypothesis), have become better known than those of our own writers, owing to their having been more effectively advertised during 1913-1918. This has caused an erroneous impression that English-speaking writers have been backward in loyal defence of Father War.

[1] Jordan (D. S.), *War and Waste*, 1913. Quoted by Maxim (Hudson), *Defenceless America* (London, New York, Toronto), p. 1.
[2] Ruskin (John), quoted by Maxim (Hudson), *Defenceless America*, (London, New York, Toronto), p. 270.

RELIGIO-THERAPEUTIC TYPE

One of the chief grievances which religious people have against those who attack their faith is generally the effect of such attacks in destroying an agreeable sense that a powerful father will do things for them, and in leaving the harsh realization that we must be our own saviours. Attacking a famous American agnostic, our friend Comstock complains :

" Ingersolism comes and says there is no help outside of man. In a recent lecture . . . one of the papers friendly to Ingersoll reports him as saying, ' I rely not upon the churches, not upon sacred books, not upon outgrown and moss-covered creeds. I rely upon human endeavour—not upon God ; I rely upon the human heart—not upon angels '."[1]
" What substitute does he offer in place of the sinner's friend ? What helps to the soul ? "[2]
" Many children are instructed in God's Word and learn by heart many precious promises. Ingersolism seeks to overthrow this saving influence."[3]
" The poor soul has tried license to do wrong and freedom to serve Satan, and realizing the results has cried out, ' Who shall deliver me from the body of this death ? '
" The scoffing lecturer replies, ' You cannot be delivered unless you do it yourself '."[4]

Closely related to the thought of the providential father is that of the father as comfortor and consoler. It is common in religion, and an example is provided in these same protests by Comstock :

" To the dying saint this scoffer cries, ' You're a fanatic, you're deluded ', and in effect says, ' The peace which passeth all understanding . . . which . . . enables you to calmly contemplate the spirit's flight from this tenement of clay, is all a delusion '."[5]

[1] Comstock (A.), *Traps for the Young* (New York, 1884), pp. 197-8.
[2] *Idem*, p. 198.
[3] *Idem*, p. 199.
[4] *Idem*, p. 203.
[5] *Idem*, p. 201.

Of the movement called Christian Science, certainly the very basis is trust in Providence. Its underlying " Principle," says Mrs Eddy, " is our Father which art in Heaven ",[1] and trust in His goodness is made the ground of the argument that all evil must be illusory. The foundress of the cult tells us that she manifested from childhood a disposition to escape from reality by satisfying her scoptophilia toward the heavenly father and so finding in him a refuge (" to seek . . . knowledge of God as . . . relief from human woe ".)[2]

Something very like Providence is certainly likewise the mainstay of New Thought and of Couéism.

New Thought

Ralph Waldo Trine is a representative of the New Thought School. His extreme expressions have called forth from one critic the remark that

" People do not exist outside of lunatic asylums and homes for inebriates who take an optimistic view on every conceivable occasion."[3]

Yet Trine continues to proclaim that :

" The optimist has the power of seeing things in their entirety and in their right relations. The pessimist looks from a limited and one-sided point of view. The one has his understanding illumined by wisdom, the understanding of the other is darkened by ignorance."[4]

[1] " What is the principle of Christian Science ? It is God, the Supreme Being, infinite and immortal Mind. . . . It is Our Father which art in Heaven." Eddy (Mrs M. A. M. B. G. P.), *Rudimental Divine Science* (Boston, 1918), p. 13.
[2] " In *Retrospection and Introspection*, Mrs Eddy says : ' From my very childhood I was impelled by a hunger and thirst after Divine things—a desire for something higher and better than matter, and apart from it—to seek diligently for the knowledge of God as the one great and ever-present relief from human woe.' " Ramsey (E. M.), *Christian Science* (Cambridge, 1924), p. 8.
[3] Bedborough (Geo.), *Harmony or Humbug* (Letchworth, 1917), p. 6.
[4] Trine (R. W.), *In Tune with the Infinite* (London, 1923), p. 1. All Trine's philosophy is founded on the trust that " the great central fact of the universe is the Spirit of Infinite Life and Power (paternal potency) behind it all." Trine (R. W.), *In Tune with the Infinite* (London, 1923), p. 3.

There is a magical technique whereby those initiated may draw good things to themselves. This consists in creating within oneself a condition " of pure delight " which reminds one of " A Case of Paranoia " commented on by Freud.[1]

The paranoiac in question recorded in his auto-biography that in order that God should continue to show him favours God demanded " a constant state of enjoyment . . . and it is my duty to provide him with this . . . in the shape of the greatest possible output of spiritual voluptuousness."[2] I hold that like the words of this paranoiac Schreber (who was lusting to be impregnated like a woman by his father) are the words of a quatrain approvingly quoted by Trine :

> " The waters know their own, and draw
> The brooks that spring in yonder height
> So flows the good with equal law
> Unto the soul of pure delight."[3]

Convinced that his attachment is reciprocated by the father, Trine is confident that the way to know, or to get, anything at all, is to go into the creator-father's sanctum (i.e. to introvert and consult conscience) and to ask him.   Trine bids us

> " Go, then, into the silence . . . and there come into contact with the Great Source of all life, of all power.   Send out your earnest desires for whatsoever you will ; and whatsoever you will, if continually watered by expectation (urethral theory of fertilization), will sooner or later come to you.   All knowledge, all truth, all power, all wisdom, all things whatsoever, are yours, if you will but go in this way for them."[4]

---

[1] Freud (S.), *Collected Papers*, transl. Strachey (London, 1925), vol. III, pp. 387-470.
[2] *Idem*, p. 415.
[3] Quoted anonymously by Trine (R. W.), *In Tune with the Infinite* (London, 1923), p. 124.
[4] Trine (R. W.), *What all the World's A-Seeking* (London, 1900), pp. 48-9.

Horatio Dresser, basing his argument upon the perfection of the intellectual and affective qualities of the father,[1] deduces that all unpleasant experiences must be only his means of leading us to ultimate benefits—especially intellectual ones[2]—and that we are therefore justified in an optimism which has no limits whatever :

> " It is a matter of economy . . . to view life and all its conditions from the brightest angle."[3]

Dresser makes it clear that the basis of this optimism is the existence of a loving father-creator behind all phenomena.

> " The omnipresent Reality, or immanent God, must love the world he has brought forth to reveal him, and therefore appreciate and love you and me as parts of it. He must have caused it to evolve from love or desire, for otherwise he would not have been compelled to cause its existence. Had he been compelled against his will, the existence of a compeller would be implied ; this is impossible, since there is but one Reality. . . . And, if he brought us here in love, he must care for our continued welfare, since he is unchangeable."[4]

His argument for the existence at all of the God in whom he believes is a most interesting bit of logic. It will be seen to amount to this : There must be what we believe in, for otherwise we have been let down, which is not Father's way of treating us.[5]

> " There must . . . be a will or purpose in this world order. For if it had no purpose, it was called forth by a non-intelligent reality, it is simply mechanical, evolution has no meaning, our desire for reasons is without a basis, and

---

[1] " In order . . . to grasp this wholeness of relationship of the great world order, let us . . . conceive this Reality as an infinitely wise, an all-loving, all-containing, all-animating Thinker." Dresser (H. W.), *Power of Silence* (London, 1898), p. 34.

[2] " Suffering then is intended to make man think." Dresser (H. W.), *Powers of Silence* (London, 1898), p. 147.

[3] *Idem*, p. 181.

[4] *Idem*, p. 46.

[5] Or the argument may be compared to the present writer contending : This thesis must be valid, for otherwise it was a mistake to have written it !

there is no reality which includes our intelligence, and we have misinterpreted nature when we deemed it the product of intelligence."[1]

Besides the narcissism which this argument reveals, it implies a view of the universe which is already closely related to providentialism. It implies that the universe would never unkindly delude us, nor let us live in false hopes.

O. S. Marden's formula for obtaining what we wish is to say to yourself frequently :

" ' All that my Father hath is mine.'—' The Lord is my shepherd I shall not want '. · If all this is true (and you know that it is) any want or lack in your life is abnormal."

" The great fundamental principle of the law of opulence is our inseparable connection with the energy of the universe. . . ."[2]

Length of life is ours also, apparently without the need of straining after hygienic living :

" It would be a reflection upon the Creator to suggest that he would limit human life to less than three times the age at which it reaches maturity (about thirty) when all the analogy of nature, especially in the animal kingdom, points to at least five times the length of the maturing period. Should not the highest manifestation of God's creation have a length of life at least equal to that of the animal ? Infinite wisdom does not shake the fruit off the tree before it is ripe."[3]

" There is not the slightest indication in the marvellous mechanism of man that he was intended to become weak, crippled and useless after a few years. A dwarfed, weak, useless man was never in the Creator's plan. . . . The Creator never made anything for retrogression ; it is

---

[1] Dresser (H. W.), *Power of Silence* (London, 1898), pp. 33-4. Again, Dresser says : " A universe must be good—that is it must fulfil a purpose, intrinsically and extrinsically, in the light of the whole and in the light of the parts—in order to exist. It must have a meaning." Dresser (H. W.), *Power of Silence* (London, 1898), p. 120.
" It must " will be seen to be simply equivalent to " I wish Father to arrange it so ".
[2] Marden (O. S.), *Peace, Power and Plenty* (New York, 1909), p. 37.
[3] Marden (O. S.), *Peace, Power and Plenty* (New York and London, 1909), p. 133.

contrary to the very nature of Deity. . . . Imagine the
Creator fashioning a man in his own likeness for only a
few years of activity."[1]

And if we ask of him for an incantation or *mantram*
to assure perpetual youth, Marden has one ready for us
which is again based on his knowledge of what must be
the providential plan :

> " Constantly affirm : ' I am always well, always young,
> I cannot grow old except by producing the old age conditions
> through my thought. The Creator intended me for con-
> tinual growth, perpetual advancement and betterment."[2]

Another adherent of the New Thought school, one not
hitherto mentioned in these pages, is the poetess, Ella
Wheeler Wilcox. Her faith in Providence is indicated
in two verses wherein she more or less identifies one's
self and one's own potency with that of the father :

> " Trust in thine own untried capacity
> As thou wouldst trust in God himself."[3]

Couéism

In the latest famous apostle of the suggestion-
therapy, I think it is clear that a very similar mentality
is at work, especially if we keep in mind what Jones
has elucidated in regard to the part played by the
father in so-called auto-suggestion. As related by an
admirer :

> " M. Coué . . . addresses himself to each one. . . .
> To the first, ' You, Monsieur, are in pain, but I tell you that
> from to-day, the cause of this pain, whether it is called
> arthritis or anything else, is going to disappear with the help
> of your unconscious . . . '

---

[1] Marden (O. S.), *Peace, Power and Plenty* (New York and London,
1909), p. 158.
" The coming man will not grow old. Perpetual youth is his destiny."
Idem, p. 159.
[2] *Idem*, p. 144.
[3] Wilcox (E. W.) : Quoted by Marden (O. S.) : *Every Man a King*
(London), p. 23.

" To the third : ' Whatever lesions you may have in your
liver, your organism is going to do what is necessary to make
the lesions disappear. . . . The bile it secretes is alkaline
and no longer acid, in the right quantity and quality.'
" M. Coué tells those present . . . ' Every morning . . .
repeat twenty times . . . counting mechanically on a
string with twenty knots in it, the following phrase :
" ' Every day, in every respect, I am getting better and
better.'
" There is no need to think of anything in particular, as
the words ' in every respect ' apply to everything."[1]

Surely the string with twenty knots in it is but the
Rosary of the Buddhist or Christian monk ! And the
trust in Providence-father is perhaps felt in the last
sentences of this quotation. Do as Coué bids, and all
will be well with us, his children, is the thought.

In this chapter, therefore, we have found that providential trust in the father has not made for realism
in the socialist or democrat, but has paved the way for
autocracy ; that it has made men over-optimistic
that war could not come or that it would result in good
and that to go to God in prayer is a substitute for self-
reliance, hard work, or medical assistance.

[1] Vs . . . oer (E.), *A Survey of the Seances,* see Coué (E), *Self
Mastery* (London, 1922), pp. 60-2.

CHAPTER V

LOYALTY

INTRODUCTORY REMARKS

" In the conservative ", says Dr M. D. Eder, " the tender tie toward the father is preserved in loyalty to the sovereign and to those persons identified with him, whilst hostility is felt toward the children (including himself) who are seeking to overthrow the father, to usurp his place, i.e. the People."[1]

As the father represents the older generation, love of the father will as a rule result in love of the ways of the older generation as opposed to those of the largely rebellious younger one. That is, the father-lovers will tend (unless the father himself should be notably progressive) towards conservatism.

This will be true in economic as well as political fields. The loving son finds it proper that the so-dear father should be in control of the family wealth. Therefore he will cavil but little at the social fathers, so to speak—the aristocracy and capitalists—being in possession of the great bulk of the country's wealth. Capitalism will seem both natural and justifiable.

Very little need be said on the subject of loyalty. We are most loyal to what we most love ; and the first objects of love are, in their order, the mother·and then the father. The son is apt to be ashamed of what he thinks an abnormally strong homosexual attachment to his father, and consequently to repress it. The accompanying loyalty will, therefore, in the degree of

---

[1] Eder (Dr M. D.), " Psycho-Analysis in Politics ", in *Social Aspects of Psycho-Analysis*, ed. by Jones (E.) (London, 1924), p. 145.

the intensity of this repression, become projected on to substitutes for the father ; for instance, on to father-like institutions.

ECONOMIC-POLITICAL TYPE

While a revolutionary movement may be motivated by hatred of the father, it seldom carries on for long without enlisting loyalty towards some new father-figure. Eder suggests that the difference in character between the French and Russian revolutions is attribut-able to the fact that the former did not so successfully as the latter substitute new fathers for old.

" The impermanency of such a revolt on the part of the band is seen in the French Reign of Terror, which offers in this particular a striking contrast with the Russian Revo-lution. . . .
" Louis XVI was executed on January 21, 1793 ; Marat was assasinated on July 13, 1793 ; Herbert was executed on March 24, 1794 ; Danton was executed April 5, 1794 ; Robespierre on July 28, 1794. . . . It is now six years since the Bolshevik revolution took place (October, 1917) and we find the original leaders still in power. I do not think any prominent Russian revolutionary leader has been assasinated or executed since the Czar was killed. Psycho-analysis offers a hint as to one factor of this difference. When I was in Russia in the winter of 1920-21, I could not help but be struck by the large number of busts of Karl Marx every-where displayed, by the prodigal array of quotations from his works. . . . What did the French revolutionists set up ? Statues of Liberty, Reason, Nature. The Russian leaders, although they had killed their father the Czar, found another father, Marx, to worship.
" The French Revolutionary leaders found no common father : as each emerged from the band in the attempt to make himself supreme leader, to become the Old Man, the Sire, the band must destroy him."[1]

[1] Eder (Dr M. D.), " Psycho-Analysis in Politics ", in *Social Aspects of Psycho-Analysis*, ed. by Jones (E.), (London, 1924), pp. 148-9.

As the father is the intellectual and executive head in most families, the *intelligenzia* are father representatives. There will, therefore, be a tendency among father-loyal persons to think the movements they are interested in, will favour the *intelligenzia*, and that the movements they opposed will be unfavourable. Equally, according as these persons feel that a movement is hospitable or hostile to intellectuals, will their father-worship make them tend to approve or disapprove of that movement.

Among the conservative faction we have Le Bon commenting on what he calls

> "Le rêve de nos socialistes modernes, d'une société d'hommes d'intelligence moyenne, d'ou toute supériorité aurait été graduellement éliminée."[1]

And Renan likewise writes :

> "Toute civilisation est l'oeuvre des aristocrates."[2]

But from the radical camp come the similarly motivated though oppositely tending accents of Bernard Shaw :

> "Social-Democracy would, in comparison, be the paradise of the able man. Every step that we make towards it takes our industry more and more out of the hands of brutes and dullards."[3]

The United States was born in a revolution. Thereafter the men who engineered this revolution came to be looked on, and even called, the fathers of the new regime. We have already touched on this and on the fact that the two most important documents which they at that time drew up have ever since been reverenced in name if not always in spirit.

---

[1] Le Bon (G.), *La Civilisation des Arabes*, 1884, p. 674. Quoted by Mallock, *Democracy*, p. iv.
[2] Renan, quoted on title page by Mallock (W. H.), *Aristocracy* (London, 1898).
[3] Shaw, *Socialism and Superior Brains* (London, 1910), p. 43.

Let us also remind the reader that one of these documents, the Declaration of Independence, is so inflammatory a resolution of revolt, that to read certain passages from it has ceased to be good form, except on Independence Day. This is especially true in times of industrial disturbance ; and persons have even been arrested for so reading.

In the other document, namely the American Constitution, there are awkward clauses, such as the free-speech amendment, which require the elaborate "interpretation" which the fatherly minds of our justices are very ready to give them. But the document as a whole enjoys a prestige remarkably like that of Holy Writ. We shall have much to say below on the irreverence of rebel sons for it, on similar irrational factors in industry, and on the constitution-worship of the conservative.

Irreverence of Socialists.

Hence it is not surprising that malcontents who show insufficient reverence to these ancient persons and documents, let themselves in for the ire of loyalists like " X——." He charges :

> " The Socialist Party . . . openly calls our constitution dishonest. It denounces the fathers of our country as grafters, as crooks, as men of mediocre intelligence, and as attorneys of the capitalist class. . . . The Socialist Party platform of 1912 explicitly demanded . . . the abolition of the United States Senate . . . of the veto power of the President . . . of the power of the Supreme Court of the United States to pass upon the constitutionality of the legislative acts ; and a revision of the constitution."
> " The Socialist Party is in particular antagonistic to the Courts."[1]

What a series of blasphemies are here indicated, indeed ! First the sacred testament of the fathers is called dishonest, then the fathers are denounced as

[1] " X——", *Is A. W. S. ?* (London, 1920), p. 18.

villains, then the assembled fathers (Senate) are to be done away with, then the supreme father (President) and father-group are symbolically to be castrated by their sacred word being revised ! It is a challenge to every drop of father-loyal blood.

Besides, the policy of these sons is so unthinkable, impossible ! One wonders what, then, save that it stirs up a personal complex, lets it so agitate him :

" If every elected and appointed officer of an American Commonwealth were to-morrow to declare himself an adherent of the socialist programme, neither he, nor all his colleagues together could do one single thing to substitute the collectivist's state for our representative democracy, save through revolution and the subversion of the constitutional principles on which our civilization and our constitution rest. . . . There is no possible way in which a socialistic state can be developed out of our representative American democracy."[1]

" X——" also accuses the Socialists of being further disloyal to the father as represented by the State. Do they not preach internationalism—*i.e.* that our own father (-land) is no better than another would be ?

" The sinister fact, never to be forgotten, about this party and its programme, is that they are . . . unpatriotic and un-American . . . America's existence is challenged."[2]

In England it is the communists who bear the full brunt of the " unpatriotic " accusation On the very breast of Mother Ocean, Mother Empire (for both are maternal symbols) is attacked by these insects :

" Great Britain is to be struck at, and if possible struck down. . . .

" We draw our life blood from the sea, and it is on the sea that we are being specially attacked. . . . Bogus blue-

---

[1] " X——", *S. W. C. O. F. of G. ?* (New York, 1912), p. 60.

[2] " Orthodox socialists are . . . anti-nationalists. . . . They desire that sort of internationalism which shall extend class consciousness, class co-operation and the class struggle beyond the boundaries of existing nations, and so assist in breaking down these boundaries. This is why the logical orthodox socialist is of necessity unpatriotic." " X——", *Is America Worth Saving ?* (London, 1920), pp. 18-9.

jackets harangue Hyde Park audiences on the alleged wrongs
of the lower decks. These men wear the name of H.M. ships
on their hat ribbons, but they belong to no British man-of-
war. They are units in that Red Armada which is being
mobilized in all the Continents for active service against
Britain. . . . The British Empire is not going to be bled to
death or even weakened by the revolutionary hornets.
The pestilent creatures can buzz and sting, but their bite is
not fatal."[1]

Communists and socialists are, however, generally
regarded by the conservative as tarred with the same
brush.[2]

But it would be wrong to imply that socialists themselves were innocent of the loyalty complex. An
instructive example to the contrary is that of H. M.
Hyndman. Faced with a schism in the ranks of the
English socialists, he recounts how

" It was quite a long time before I understood why the
Fabians went away from us . . . ' It seems quite incredible to me,' I said, ' that they cannot see that Marx's
analysis is perfectly correct . . . I don't like to accuse them
of intellectual dishonesty—— '

" ' I do ' was the reply . . . They saw that if they
accepted Marx's teachings they merely followed . . . you
social democrats in the footsteps of a great genius by whom
they would . . . be over-shadowed . . .

" Years later . . . I agreed to address what is called the
' Fabian Nursery ' on Karl Marx's theories . . . They knew
it all . . . beforehand . . . and what they did, not know
was not worth knowing.

[1] *Daily Mail*, August 24th. . . . Quoted in *New Leader* (for ridicule),
(London, August 28th, 1925).
[2] " The distinction between the Hamburg International and the
Third International of Moscow is merely that one might be described
as the right wing and the other the left wing of the same movement.
Indeed, the former has refused to condemn the methods of the latter ;
it realises well enough that they cannot afford to quarrel. Both are
engaged in the work of overthrowing the present social system. Why
quarrel with your neighbour merely because he does it in a different
way ? Similarly, the British Socialist party has found it impossible
to exclude communists from their party." Northumberland, in introduction to Mallock, *Democracy* (London, 1924), p. xi.
It is only fair to say this was written before September 29th, 1925,
when, at the Labour Conference, the exclusion of Communists from
the British Labour Party was made absolute by an enormous
majority.—P.H.

" A young man had cultivated an air of æsthetic boredom and elegant inanity . . . ' I never read any of Marx,' he said . . . The next speaker was younger still ; he had ' read Marx many years ago, but really had forgotten all about it ! ' A nursery indeed !

" Then I went down to Cambridge to address the Fabian Society there . . . who, however, confessed themselves that they had never taken the trouble to master the theories upon which the whole international socialist movement is based. They, too, patronized Marx, talked of him as ' not up-to-date ', and tried to impress me with the vast superiority of some unknown gods of political economy . . . Sunk in the Jevonian bog I found them."[1]

There is, in all this, an astonishing approach to the attitude of the good elder son, who has stepped into his father's shoes to upbraid his less respectful brothers for a breach of filial piety. We suspect that Marx became, for Hyndman, a surrogate for the more loved portion of his father-*imago*.

If so, it was natural that the new world of greater social justice which, for Marx, this new father, took the place of the house and land in which he once had lived— that this new home, this new Fatherland of the Socialist Commonwealth, should be adopted as his own by Hyndman, and should be regarded by him as a perfect heaven. In this paradise, as a matter of course, beauty —or *art*—should maternally queen it, freed from such things as hamper her under the capitalism that Marx demanded.

But to the anti-socialist, the obstacles to an ideal fatherland here below seem too great. So if he be a religious man, he prefers to posit paradise as a place or state to be attained only after death. In general, too, the conception of paradise as having its *locus* above the clouds carries the paternal sanction of old tradition. An example of opposition to Socialism on such theological grounds is given in the *Anti-Socialist Speaker's Hand-book :*

[1] Hyndman (H. M.), *Further Reminiscences* (London, 1912), pp. 214-6.

" Socialism encourages men and women to seek their
satisfaction in this life . . . Professor Ferri says, ' Socialism
. . . tends to substitute itself for religion, because it desires
precisely that humanity should have in itself its own " ter-
restrial paradise ", without having to wait for it in a " something beyond ", which, to say the least, is very problemati-
cal '. Professor Karl Pearson declares, ' Socialism arises
from the recognition that the sole aim of mankind is happiness in this life '. . . This is the kind of teaching that
filters down from the thinkers and writers to the rank and
file ."[1]

" The moral, therefore, is plain. If . . . religion and
the churches are worth saving, Socialism must be resisted."[2]

Northumberland, also, finds that the movement
threatens the worship of the Heavenly Father :

" What is this great movement, after all, but a combined
attack on civilization by the forces of subversion, pro-
fessing a creed which denies all the implications of Christian
civilization ? . . .

" Those who are sincerely desirous to better the lot of
their fellows . . . are the dupes, and their fate is always
to be submerged by their followers, who are deterred by no
scruples and who are actuated only by the terrible logic
of the fanatic."[3]

Of the Christian Socialist another critic says :

" It may also be asked which view of human life he is
prepared to adopt : the Christian view, which makes this
life entirely subordinate to the next, regarding pain and
suffering as the means by which we are perfected and fitted
for a heavenly state of existence ; or the socialist view,
which regards pain and suffering as an unmitigated curse,
and a happy social life, amidst ease and comfort, as the
chief object of human existence ? "[4]

Nor does " X——" refrain from adding *his* warning,
which is based on the conception that all human goodness
began with the Father of our religion, and will die out

---

[1] *Anti-Socialist Union Speakers' Handbook* (London, 1911), p. 210.
[2] *Idem*, p. 221.
[3] Northumberland, in introduction to Mallock (W. H.), *Democracy*
(London, 1924), p. xii.
[4] *Anti-Socialist Union Speakers' Handbook* (London, 1911), pp. 26-7.

when the general father-revering attitude of the community diminishes :

> "The American people may . . . install a collectivist or socialist state, but . . . they will starve to death those splendid traits of benevolence, human kindness and charity which have marked . . . civilization since the religion of Christ became one of its most potent moving forces."[1]

Naturally, when it comes to communism, the case is infinitely worse. The sacrileges of the Bolsheviks have sent a shudder of horror through all father-loyal Christendom :

> "Moscow committed another blasphemy, we are told, when the city recently dedicated a child to communism at a ' civil christening ' at which Isadora Duncan and a number of children danced to the strains of ' Ave Maria ' . . . The child, daughter of peasant parents, was accepted by the aged ' priestess ' of the Red International, Klara Zetkin, and by Bukharin, one of the executive committee, who was himself ' aflame with devotion to Russia's new religion '. So, comments the Cincinnati *Enquirer*, ' In a great theatre, before an immense audience of the faithful who deny God, a little child, clothed in red, in the arms of a revolutionary assassin, was dedicated to the cause of Communism."[2]

Especially will the new doctrines undermine those virtues which we particularly associate with the fathers— those which have to do with the accumulation and turning over to us of property. The time when the father was a rival or competitor was very long ago. He has since become, says " X——," our hero, our *super ego* " with a moral purpose " :

> "That which the American of to-day opposes to socialist autocracy is not the crude competitive individualism of the old-fashioned economist, but co-operative individualism with a moral purpose . . . On the existence of private capital . . . depend the virtues of thrift, of liberality and of sacrifice."[3]

---

[1] " X——", *S. W. C. O. F. of G ?* (New York, 1912), p. 61.
[2] Abstracted in *The Literary Digest* (New York, December 29th, 1923).
[3] " X——", *Is A. W. S. ?* (London, 1920), p. 22.

At various times and places does " X—— " stress
the altruistic motive which lies behind the institution,
of the fathers. In the following passage he makes
this a reason why the fatherland must decline to perceive
the fact of a distinction between fathers and sons.
Speaking of " inalienable rights " of acquiring, possessing
and protecting property, he says :

> " Their basis is a moral one. What American civilization
> is striving to do is to give moral persons full opportunity
> for their most complete development and expression. For
> this fundamental reason America cannot tolerate the notion
> of fixed or definite economic classes, that have conflicting
> interests."[1]

Another representative of the father is the king.
Inevitably, therefore, the rebellious socialist sons become
suspect of plotting against the father in this form as well
as in others. And even as civilization is to fall with
Father Christ, and morality, benevolence, etc., are to
decay with Father Capitalism, so justice must crumple
with Father Royalty :

> " The first action of a socialist government will be to
> abolish the Crown and proclaim a Socialist Common-
> wealth."[2]
> " It is difficult to conceive what objection any socialist
> can have to a monarch whose rule is one of wisdom and
> beneficence.[3]
> " The King is the embodiment of justice."

Irrational Factors in Industry

The treatment of property rights as more sacred than
human rights—seen in instances where employers interfere with passing or carrying out regulations intended
to protect men from dangerous machinery, or women or
children from excessive hours—is thus the triumph of
father over son. When Robert Owen endeavoured to

[1] " X—— ", *Is A. W. S. ?* (London, 1920), pp. 20-21.
[2] *Anti-Socialist Union Speakers' Handbook* (London, 1911), p. 150.
[3] *Idem*, p. 151.

persuade other employers to imitate the reforms he had
introduced into his mills at Lanark, he laid before them
convincing evidence that the reforms had redounded to
his own profit. In spite of this, he persuaded no one.
Their Œdipus complexes against the employees (sons)
were apparently stronger than their love of gain. For :

"That irrational elements are present in capitalism
is shown not only in the discussions on currency, but in
every commercial transaction, in the very conception of
succession, in the accumulation of large fortunes."[1]

This irrationality increases immensely the difficulty
of understanding the other man's point of view. Many
Socialists credit the Capitalists of all the world with
conspiring against them with a cunning which, if it
existed, would be hopeless for the former to contend
against, any more than the child can hope to contend
against his father. Sometimes the conservative is
similarly frightened by rumours of conspiracies and
" protocols " among the sons. At other times, swinging
towards a contempt of his opponents that is equally
extreme (and arguing in the present case somewhat in a
circle, through excess of affect) he charges :

"Socialists of all schools are socialists because they are
ignorant of . . . principles of nature and of human nature.
. . . They could not be socialists unless they were thus

[1] Further : " Capitalism has as one of its main supports the infant's
pleasure in its bodily functions, and the reaction-formations caused by
the proper demands of education. . . . That . . . these tendencies
may be of first rate political importance is seen in the financial policy
of rapid deflation which this country has adopted. You have but to
read some of the recent speeches for and against the deflation to opine
that there must be some other motives than those given making the idea
of a gold standard so full of horror or so attractive. The *New Statesman*,
in a note on the subject in a recent issue, seems to have guessed the
secret. The writer says that : ' The Policy of the abandonment of
deflation is obscured at present by excited controversialists who throw
about the words inflation and deflation like stink bombs. . . .'
" It is worth noting that, generally speaking . . . the bankers and
the financiers, those who deal in money, are the powerful adherents of
deflation, while the industrialists tend to disfavour rapid deflation,
for they have, as a class, found substitutes for the primitive analerotic
wishes." *Social Aspects of Psycho-Analysis*, ed. by Jones (E.), (London,
1924), pp. 165-6.

ignorant. In this they resemble the devisers of . . .
infallible systems for breaking the bank at a roulette-
table."[1]

The reader will recall certain citations in Part I, from
Hyndman and Shaw, of which the symbollic sense was,
that no child's pocket money should be held back because
the child's nature happened to be one of laziness or
naughtiness. This represented an extreme position.
Yet it does correspond to a general tendency among
socialists to exculpate the individual and blame circumstances. Nothing, they say—thus far with science—
is uncaused. Look to the environment, or that plus
heredity, add the broader-minded, and you will understand why the individual is what he is. Blame his
Creator and, above all, blame the one who disciplines,
teaches or starves him, namely Society (father again)
but do not blame the poor lad himself whom these have
produced. If he is stunted, it is because Institutions
(father) have robbed him of Mother Nature's milk.

Against which, " X—— " thunders a defence of
the fathers (corporation ; business) :

" Our troubles do not arise from the size of corporations,
they do not arise from the percentage of control of business
. . . they arise not from limited liability corporations at
all, no matter how big they are ; but . . . from individual
delinquents ; and we need no more law than we have now
to get at individuals who commit immoral offences, dis-
honourable acts."[2]

It is important to notice that loyalty to the father,
while it generally makes for conservatism, does not work
out that way invariably. Some, indeed, of our socialists

---

[1] Mallock (W. H.), *Critical Examination of Socialism* (London, 1908)
p. 163.
[2] " X—— ", *S. W. C. O. F. of G. ?* (New York, 1912), p. 84.
Doubtless, " X—— " here expresses an intuitive sense of the anti-
paternal motive which is present in so much of law-breaking.
" Hostility toward the father . . . is a partial explanation of smug-
gling, of evading the income tax, of cheating company, etc." Eder
(Dr M. D.), " Psycho-Analysis in Politics ", in *Social Aspects of Psycho-
Analysis*, ed. by Jones (E.), (London, 1924), p. 154.

would almost seem to agree with " X——" as far as
punishing the individual is concerned ; they doubtless
are in a minority, but what a loyal son of the paternal
state we have in Karl Pearson, who is arguing not against
socialism, mind you, but *for* it :

> " Socialists have to inculcate that spirit which would
> give offenders against the state short shrift and the
> nearest lamp-post.   Every citizen must learn to say
> with Louis XIV, *L'état c'est moi*."[1]

Certainly this statement would damn the movement
with any but father-sympathizers, if generally supported !
A more moderate and, fortunately, more widely accepted
expression of the father-attitude, is seen when

> " The Fabian Society resolutely opposes all pretensions
> to hamper the socialization of industry with equal wages,
> equal hours of labour, equal official status, or equal authority
> for everyone."[2]

What seems an unusually naïve implication that sons
exist in order that fathers may exploit them, is found in
an argument against free trade on the score that it

> " takes from the middle classes the source from which their
> servants were obtained ; it practically abolishes the class of
> most value as emigrants to British colonies."[3]

Finally, one writer tries to make his point by means
of the following confused analogy, in which the only
thing clearly evident appears to be a desire that things
be paternally regulated :

> " It is not the entire absence of restraint that gives the
> citizen freedom to move about his streets as he chooses,
> but the restraining force of police and penal laws . . . So
> it is in matters of foreign trade."[4]

---

[1] Pearson (Prof. Karl), *Ethics of Free Thought*, p. 324.   Quoted by
Anti-Socialist Speakers' Handbook, p. 18.
[2] *Report on Fabian Policy*, Tract no. 70, p. 7.   Quoted by *Anti-
Socialist Speakers' Handbook*, p. 72.
[3] Williams (E. E.), *Case for Protection* (London, 1899), p. 36.
[4] *Idem*, p. 36.

Constitution-Worship

Various psycho-analytic writers have commented on the manner in which loyalty to the father may become displaced on to the head of the state or even on to the state itself.[1]

Eder makes the following comment on

> " Blackstone's well-known formula : ' The sovereign is not only incapable of doing wrong, but even of thinking wrong ; he can never mean to do an improper thing ; in him is no folly or weakness.' Put briefly, it is the maxim that the king can do no wrong, and its genesis is : My father can do no wrong."[2]

Most men to-day are astonished that such words as those of Blackstone could have been uttered by a man of his parts. Yet I find a more modern controversialist to proclaim :

> " Our constitution . . . is acknowledged to be the most perfect in the world, and of it . . . the monarchy is the first essential . . . It is ideal government for Britons."[3]

It can next be shown how these same sentiments can still be expressed when nominally more democratic symbols have replaced those of sovereign, king and monarchic constitution. For this I shall refer to two books by " X—— ". And first I would have the reader note how the theme of loyalty to the father is expressly set forth on the dedicatory pages :

> " To the memory of my father and mother, gentlefolk of

---

[1] " In the displacement of the father-regarding feeling on to the state, the tendencies connected with the attitude of respect, obedience and loyalty to the paternal authority are usually the most prominent. Great importance is, moreover, almost invariably attached to the head of the state as its embodiment and its supreme authority, the country over which he rules being looked upon as his possession or estate, which it is the duty of his children to uphold, to protect or to enlarge." Flügel (J. C.), *Psycho-Analytic Study of the Family*, 1921, p. 126.

[2] Eder (Dr M. D.), " Psycho-Analysis in Relation to Politics ", in *Social Aspects of Psycho-Analysis*, ed. by Jones (E.), (London, 1924), p. 187.

[3] *Anti-Socialist Union Speakers' Handbook* (London, 1911), p. 151.

the old school who taught their sons to care for the public affairs and to follow high standards in doing so."[1]

This we read, in the one book ; and the dedication of the second is equivalent in purport :

> "To all those Americans who . . . have faith in those ideals . . . which the fathers have conceived."[2]

We ought by this to be suitably prepared for the panegyrics upon native American Institutions which follow, and which so interestingly parallel the one cited above on British institutions. This man, whose position constitutes him an authority, rhapsodises :

> "Never in the history of the world, before or since, has there been displayed so much insight into the principles of government, so much knowledge of the theory and practical workings of the different forms of government, as that which accompanied the formulation and adoption of the constitution of the United States. Truly, there were giants in those days."[3]

That was in the earlier book. After the war (during which "red" sons were mobbed or arrested by conservatives for merely reading so inflammatory a document as the Declaration of Independence), this conservative writer is nevertheless still found loyal to it, as a paternal scripture :

> "The Declaration of Independence rings as true to-day as it did in 1776. The constitution remains the surest and safest foundation for a free government that the wit of man has yet devised."[4]

---

[1] "X——", *W. S. W. C. O. F. of G. ?* (New York, 1912). Dedicatory page.

[2] "X——", *Is A. W. S. ?* (London, 1920). Dedicatory page.

[3] "X——", *W. S. W. C. O. F. of G. ?* (New York, 1912), pp. 6-7.
One cannot help remarking that it must have been a great blow to this panegyrist that not a single one of the new nations created by the great war chose to model its constitution after that of the United States.

[4] "X——", *Is A. W. S. ?* (London, 1920), p. 24.

Finally, we can again cite " X——" as maintaining the merits of certain political forms, on the score that they have been peculiar to our own race, which has brought them forth from hoary antiquity :

" The fundamental principles underlying our constitutional government, our representative democracy, are those which are the product of the settled habits of thinking of the Anglo-Saxon race. It took many hundreds of years and countless struggles to discover and to establish them."[1]

HUMANITARIAN TYPE

We have seen that love of the fatherland means love of the father. To be unpatriotic is an unforgivable sin. The region in which the father has elected to dwell is associated with his personality. The child's reaction to the flag under which his father fought and to the nationality and country which were his, becomes conditioned by feelings originally directed to the father himself. So the children come to speak of their *father*-land (as well as of the *mother*-country). Sentiments of loyalty displaced from him on to the nation are significantly called *pat*riotism. Themselves are *pat*riots.

Moreover, as one reads what militaristic writers say about the benefits of war, one becomes convinced that many of them secretly feel what Heraclitus explicitly said :

" War is the father of all things."[2]

Add to this that the father can do no wrong, and such loyalty readily explains some of the statements, so completely in contradiction to human experience, which the sons of Mars are continually making. They crop up

[1] " X——", *W. S. W. C. O. F. of G. ?* (New York, 1912), p. 60.
[2] Heraclitus, as quoted by Maxim (Hudson), *Defenceless America* (London, New York, Toronto), p. 272.

even in the writings of pretended economists. Take for example this piece of puerility :

"Military expenditure . . . as far as it goes to British subjects, is but a transfer of value . . . Taxes paid to British subjects, are but a transfer of value."[1]

On the other hand, loyalty to the father sometimes operates as a factor in pacifism. Thus, some persons find in the example, if not in the explicit teachings of their prophet or religious father such as Buddha or Jesus, something which they fancy to be incongruous with faith in the cutting of throats as a final arbitrament. Or it may be that these persons are influenced by an actually living father or father-substitute thus to idealize peacefulness and hate violence. In the case of Tolstoy, who was one of the two most famous of modern non-resistants, and inspirer of the other one (Gandhi) this influence was exerted through an elder brother, a figure that frequently takes the father rôle. (Leof Tolstoy's real father died when Leof was very small).[2] Tolstoy thereafter became spiritual father to Ghandi, that Hindu pacifist who has had more followers than any moral leader ever before had in his own life-time.

RELIGIO-THERAPEUTIC TYPE

Following the fashion of all early religions, Pythagoras included among his precepts :

"Honour thy parents and kinsfolk."[3]

[1] Byles (J. B.), *Sophisms of Free Trade* . . . *Exposed* (London and New York, 1904), pp. 127-8.

[2] "At the age of five, Tolstoy's imagination was fired by his brother telling him of a green stick, buried at the edge of a ravine, on which was written the secret which would make all men happy and enable them to live in loving harmony with one another, free from pain, sorrow, anger, or distress. Tolstoy's life—especially the last thirty years of it— was devoted to the discovery of that magic message, and to communicating what he could decipher of it to mankind." Maude (Aylmer), *Leo Tolstoy* (London, 1918), p. 5.

[3] Quoted from the "Golden Words", by Harrison (F.), *New Calendar* (London, 1922), p. 107.

In almost the same phraseology (hinting at an identity of underlying meaning), he likewise commands :

" Honour the deathless gods, as the law (word of the father) ordains."[1]

Accordingly, it would be disloyal to question the perfection or set limits to the potency of the fathers.

" Disbelieve nothing wonderful concerning the gods, nor concerning divine dogmas."[2]

An equally obvious attachment to the fathers, to the words they spoke as being wise and to the conduct they enjoined as being good, and an inhibition against invoking their name (oaths) is found in the case of the Essenes. According to the account given by Philo :

" It is ethics to which they devote all their strength, under the guidance of their ancestral laws, which no human soul could have devised apart from ancestral inpirations.

" In these laws they are instructed, particularly on the seventh day, as well as at other times. For the seventh day is held sacred ; on it they cease all constructive work, and repair to sacred places called synagogues, where they sit arranged, according to age—young below the older persons —and listen with due order and attention.

" One reads aloud the sacred books . . . They are taught piety, holiness . . . Thus they furnish thousands of examples of the meaning of love of God, by a close and continuous purity maintained throughout life, by abstinence from oaths and falsehood, and by regarding the deity as the cause of all good but no evil."[3]

Among the Sufi sect of *Mevlevees*, loyalty to the order, its founder and other father-figures is tested out by an apprenticeship of 1001 days.[4] Curiously enough this

---

[1] Quoted from the " Golden Words," by Harrison (F.), *New Calendar* (London, 1922), p. 107.
[2] *Pythagorean Symbols With Explanations by Iamblicus.* Trans. Bridgman, p. 68.
[3] Philo., *Quod Omnis Probus Liber. G* 12. Quoted by Moffatt (J.), in art. " Essenes ", in *Encyclopædia of Religion and Ethics.*
[4] " ' How does one become a dervish ? ' I asked. " By long apprenticeship. Perhaps our order (the Mevlevees) has the most severe novitiate. The candidate must labour as a male servitor of the lowest rank for 1001 days before he can be received, during which time he is called the karra kohals (jackal). For one day's failure he has to begin

sect required the candidate to report his dreams to the
Sheik of the order, although whether the latter resolves
the transference in anything like psycho-analytic fashion
is more doubtful. Dr MacGovern and others told me
that in certain Buddhist monasteries the abbot likewise requires dreams to be brought to him.

Although father-loyalty may be found in anti-
religious persons,[1] it more commonly brings about a
pro-religious attitude, and a hostility to atheists and
agnostics. The arguments of the latter, and especially
any witticisms they make at the expense of theology,
are resented, just as personal affronts to one's own
father would be. Comstock is an illustration of the loyal
son thus shocked :

> " Every person must respect the infidel who says ' I
> cannot see nor understand these matters of religion as you
> do, I wish I could '. There is a vast difference between
> such an one and the one who scoffs and sneers, or makes a
> living by blaspheming the name of God.
> " If newspaper reports and the printed speeches of
> Mr Ingersoll are to be credited, his forte is to discuss the
> weightiest and most solemn subjects so as to provoke from
> his audience ' laughter ', ' loud laughter ', ' shouts of
> laughter ', and ' applause '."[2]
> " The liberal leaders . . . loudly blaspheme the name
> of God, and seem to take special delight in printing God,
> Lord, or Jesus Christ, commencing each with small letters
> . . . Sabbath laws they seek to . . . abrogate." [3]

again from the beginning. There are particular phrases, too, that
he must repeat in retirement hundreds of times a day and report to the
Sheik of the order the dreams that may have occurred to him. They
are the same phrases that the law requires all true dervishes to repeat
each day, for it is by such invocation of God that the breath of man
becomes holy and acquires superior power." Cornwall (Ruth), " Whirling Doctors of Divinity ", *New York Times Magazine*, July 15th, 1923.
    [1] Huxley (Prof. T. H.), p. 127. Thus Huxley offers the following
tribute to Mr Wharton Jones :—
" The extent and precision of his knowledge impressed me greatly,
and the severe exactness. . . . I do not know that I have ever felt
so much respect for anybody before or since. I worked hard to obtain
his approbation, and he was extremely kind and helpful to the youngster
who, I am afraid, took more of his time than he had any right to."
    [2] Comstock (A.), *Traps for the Young* (New York, 1884), p. 184.
    [3] *Idem*, p. 197.

When he thinks of these rebel sons, Comstock's blood boils, and in his loyalty to the Heavenly Father, he projects unto them certain qualities such as inconsistency, narrowness and distortion of facts which were, as his own records shows, outstanding traits of our crusader himself :

" Their crude and narrow views they parade above the wisdom and learning of scholars. They put their leader— the great American blasphemer—before God.

" The experience and teachings of good men of all ages go for naught. They are inconsistent, arrogant, narrow-minded and bigotted ; fierce and violent against all who differ from them. Lying and deceit are their stronghold. To distort facts is their glory.

" To assault their enemies in an underhanded and base manner, and take every advantage over those they oppose is their peculiar delight."[1]

Let us now pass from the discussion of Comstock to a consideration of Quimby and of Mrs Eddy as regards this loyalty-complex.

Quimby

We saw how the Essenes regarded the father as the *cause of all good but no evil.* Quimby reached this identical state of reverence, and added the logical loyal corrollary, that it is always the sons who are at fault.

" The foundation of his theory, regarded simply as a belief is, that disease is not self existent, nor created by God, but is purely an invention of man."[2]

---

[1] More recently a divine, Dr Davidson, voices as follows his loyalty to the sayings and beliefs of the fathers :—
" We do well to say the old creed, to uplift the familiar, the well-proven prayers. The phrases, though cast in other days, other surroundings than ours, and retaining their birthmarks, are no empty survival of effete or dying things ; they live. They have hands and feet. Of course, it is true that here, of anywhere on earth, we are in touch with sacred things of old. We are in touch with Him who liveth and was dead, with Him who is Omega as well as Alpha, with Him who hath—not had—the keys." Quoted by Lloyd (J. T.), in *Free-thinker* (London, July 16th, 1925).
[2] *The Free Press,* Lebanon, Me., December 3rd, 1860 ; quoted by Dresser (A. G.), *Philosophy of P. P. Quimby* (Boston, 1895), p. 28.

For it is axiomatic with him that the father—of whom wisdom is classically the attribute, and whom only Quimby can mean when he speaks of wisdom as though it were a person—that the father, I say, can contain no imperfection and intend no evil.

> " Wisdom contains no opinion or selfishness, and, like charity, has no illwill towards its neighbour, but like the rays of the sun, is always ready to impart heat to all who will come to the light."[1]

It is usual to speak of the heavenly father as being everywhere and permeating everything. Quimby uses the same language with regard to wisdom, thus confirming our premise that with him father and wisdom are synonyms :

> " God is not matter, and matter is only an idea that fills no space in wisdom, and as wisdom fills all space, all ideas are in wisdom."[2]

Indeed, he finally declares the identification in so many words :

> " My God is wisdom, and all wisdom is of God ; where there is no wisdom there is no God."[3]

The patients of P. P. Quimby seem to have felt great loyalty toward their teacher and physician. Apparently his character was such as to elicit their tenderest father-associations. One of them testifies :

> " The sick person, who is like one cast into prison for an unjust deed, can feel the force of his system. With a sympathy which the sick alone can call forth, and a knowledge which he proves alone to them, he leads an invalid along the path to health. His power over disease comes from subtle knowledge of mind . . . to which subject his mind was turned some twenty years ago by mesmerism."[4]

---

[1] Quimby (P. P.), see Dresser (H.W.), *Quimby Manuscripts* (London), p. 184.
[2] *Idem*, p. 408.
[3] *Idem*, p. 408.
[4] H — (a patient of Quimby), in *The Advertiser* (Portland, Me., February, 1860).

Mrs Eddy

The loyalty which his followers felt towards Quimby, one of them, when she founded a new church upon his teaching, deflected partly to herself,[1] and partly to the new scriptures which she penned. The precautions to be observed in the presence of the sacred text of the cult, lest it should be defiled, are most interesting :

> " No objectionable pictures shall be exhibited in the rooms where the Christian Science Textbook is published or sold. No idle gossip, no slander, no evil speaking shall be allowed."[2]

The identification of wisdom with the father, made by Quimby, was carried on by his pupil, with at times slight changes of language. At one time she prays :

> " May Christ, Truth, be present."

Elsewhere we find this :

> " God is the Principle of Metaphysical Science . . . God is a Principle."[3]

This seems to mean that Mrs Eddy deified that attribute of her father which, to her as a child, seemed most characteristic of him—he stood for the embodiment of an abstraction, Truth.

To recapitulate some points of this chapter ; the loyalty which first was directed to the father may become displaced onto Karl Marx, superior men, an ideal fatherland, Loyalty, the State, the national constitution or institutions, an elder brother as with Tolstoy, gods, ancestors, a holy book, Christ or truth.

---

[1] So that it becomes necessary to decree that " A member of the Mother Church shall not haunt Mrs Eddy's drive when she goes out, continually stroll by her house, or make a summer resort near her for such a purpose." Eddy (Mrs M. A. M. B. G. P.), *Church Annual* (Boston, 1924), p. 43.

[2] *Idem*, p. 81.

[3] Eddy (Mrs M. A. M. B. G. P.), *The Science of Man*, 1876, p. 5.

CHAPTER VI

AUTHORITY, CONFORMITY, SUGGESTION, AND AUTO-SUGGESTION

Introductory Remarks

THE child is drilled into continual submission to the *dicta* of its parents. When the parents command, the child must obey or suffer withdrawal of love which it craves. When the parents make a prediction or venture an opinion, this is generally found to be justified by future events, to a degree which impresses the child. Many parents, besides, are given to harping on their own infallibility. From these facts arise the closely related phenomena of authority, conformity, suggestion and auto-suggestion.

Authority

In course of time parental pretensions, like other forms of charlatanry, come to be found out. But habits of obedience and respect are deeply ingrained. Where the habits refer to the parent of like sex with the child they derive unrecognized reinforcement from repressed components of homosexuality.

This tendency to rely upon the pronouncements of superiors, therefore, is often found in children to whom the parents have never been excessively severe.[1]

---

[1] " A child who never disobeyed his parents and who never felt their authority as irksome would in all likelihood be sadly deficient in individuality and initiative in later life. For this reason the arousal of a desire to rebel against the parents (with the accompanying feelings of hostility) is not in every case to be condemned." Flügel (J. C.), *Psycho-Analytic Study of the Family*, p. 188.

Those whom we love we seek to please by following in the paths of conduct they have indicated for us. So the rules laid down by a deceased loved father become binding upon us and tend to allay many of the hostile feelings we harboured toward him during his life, by placing him where he can do nothing to arouse jealousy. After his death, therefore, the love for our father binds us in some respects, more, rather than less, than before.

Dead, the father becomes our ancestor. The ancestors, the ancients, as it were, take him unto themselves. As he himself is now only a memory, it is the easier for us to transfer some of the love and respect we felt for him, to them as a class.

All those who naturally become father-surrogates, of course, gain by the reverence in which the central figure himself has been held. Brother (especially if elder brother), teacher, able man, aristocrat, admired person or class, the state (in state worship) and the authorities in various fields, are gainers.

The facts above alluded to give rise to what Miss Bradbury has called The Fallacy of Authority:

> "A tendency to accept 'authority' instead of forming independent judgment, as illustrated, for instance, in the savage's proneness to rely on tribal custom or upon the word of medicine man, priest, or king, or by the tendency among civilized men to base arguments upon the authority of religious creeds or the dogmas of scientific textbooks; this fallacy (like all the subsequent ones) appearing in its most insidious form when the real basis of the argument is unrecognized, e.g. when a man thinks he is arguing from purely scientific premises, but is all the time being unconsciously influenced by a religious bias.
> "It is obvious that a more penetrating analysis of the psychological mechanism of this form of fallacy would deal with the nature of our attitude towards parents and parent-substitutes."[1]

---

[1] Bradbury (M. K.), *The Logic of the Unconscious Mind*, as reviewed by Flügel (J. C.), in *The International Journal of Psycho-Analysis*, vol. II (London, 1921), p. 126.

Conformity

A phenomenon related to authority as negative to positive is that of conformity. The individual, instead of striking out a path for himself, is content to take his lead from the group which has father-like prestige. MacCurdy evinces an insight into the operation of this trait :

> " If contrast and relative incompatibility between intelligence and conformity exist, it would only be reasonable to infer that the latter is an instinctive phenomenon. And, indeed, these manifestations do show in a fairly complete way the three characteristics which Rivers points out for instincts. They tend to follow the ' all or none ' law. A middle ground is hard to hold. One cannot agree with a solid group of people . . . and preserve independent judgment . . . Second . . . these phenomena are unreflective or they are nothing. The third, that of the reaction being immediate or uncontrolled, holds true when the instinct is expressed in a reaction rather than a motivation. There are few kinds of conduct less immediate and controlled than the pillaging of a mob. During war all our enemies are inhuman monsters."[1]

Bertrand Russell says :

> " What we ' ought ' to desire is merely what someone else wishes us to desire. Usually it is what the authorities wish us to desire—parents, schoolmasters, policemen, and judges."[2]

All these persons, the reader will note, are paternal surrogates. In the United States the source of ultimate authority, beyond even the President or Congress, is the Supreme Court, in which is vested the interpretation of the political scriptures. No less an authority than that of these holy fathers is invoked by Comstock to sanction his way of imposing morality upon America :

---

[1] MacCurdy, *Dynamic Psychology* (London, 1923), pp. 324-5.
[2] Russell (B.), " The Good Life ", in *What I Believe* (London, 1925), pp. 37-8.

" The Supreme Court of the United States approves and sanctions the very method which has been pursued by the writer from the beginning."[1]

Suggestion

Next, let us take up the much-mooted topic of conformity of the very will itself to a loved or feared authority, namely, suggestion. As we have previously seen, there are two methods of producing hypnosis. One is the quiet, pleading manner. This we found to correspond to infantile experience of the lulling, soothing mother, and, therefore, it does not come within the scope of this essay. The other method, the authoritative one, will alone detain us.

As the father is the authority and command-giver in most families, so it is that one half or more of hypnotic practice is based on the hypnotist establishing himself in the father's place in the subject's thought. Rapport consists in doing that. This matter has been very thoroughly thrashed out by psycho-analytic writers, and I shall, therefore, only express a conclusion, formed after some experience of my own in this field,[2] of agreement with the view of the psycho-analytic school on the nature of will,[3] hypnotism and suggestion. Following the lead, especially, of Ernest Jones, who has made such a splendid examination of the matter,[4] I also concur in the idea that so-called auto-suggestion is only a special

[1] Comstock (A.), *Traps for the Young* (New York, 1884), p. 237.

[2] See Hopkins (P.), *A Study of Motivation*, a thesis accepted in partial fulfillment of the requirement for the degree of M.A. at Teacher's College of Columbia University, New York, 1910.

[3] " Without wishing to embark on a discussion of the nature of will, I may briefly state my agreement with Lipp's view that the sense of will, and of striving or effort altogether, really emanates from a consciousness of inhibition, or—put in more modern language—an intuition that in respect of the idea in question the conscious ego is inhibiting other unconscious, mental processes. At all events it is plain that the will is specially connected with the conscious ego, and particularly the ego ideal." Jones (E.), " The Nature of Auto-Suggestion ", *The International Journal of Psa.* (London, 1923), vol. IV.

[4] See Jones (E.), " The Nature of Auto-Suggestion ", *The International Journal of Psa.* (London, 1923), vol. IV.

form of hetero-suggestion, in which the doctor[1] or some-one else is still present to recall the authority of the father, and in which, furthermore, the ego-ideal which is invoked in the act of self-suggesting is itself largely modelled upon the subject's early ideals of the father.

The employment by many hypnotists of what we may call shock or surprise tactics, may serve me now as a means of transition to the topic of the intriguingness of the marvellous. William James long ago spoke of " the vertiginous fascination " of even unpleasant things, when, e.g. one went on smelling again a disagreeable odour just to see how bad it really was.

This has caused Miss Bradbury to enumerate as among those dangers to clear thinking on which I have quoted her one she calls the Fallacy of the Marvellous :

" A tendency to believe in a thing because it is marvellous ; as illustrated by our readiness to make a nine days' wonder out of anything which offers possibilities (such as the case of Helen Keller) or our alacrity in spreading and believing reports of supernatural phenomena. A full treatment of the psychological causes of this fallacy would have to deal with, among other things, (1) The intellectual basis of the fallacy in limitation or dissociation of experience (an aspect already treated by McDougall and other psychologists) ; (2) The belief in magic and the supernatural generally as arising from a projection of the primitive " omnipotence of thought " ; (3) The narcissistic roots of the motives leading to exaggeration as a means of increasing the power and interest attaching to the individual (a matter on which psycho-analytic research has still probably much enlighten-ment to give us.)"[2]

[1] " Clinically every physician who endeavours to teach his patients how to use auto-suggestion, as I did myself some 20 years ago, will probably be able to confirm my experience of finding how very hard it is to estimate the importance of the part played by the idea of the physician in the patients' mind, and to distinguish between this and the other factors at work. The gradation between hetero- and auto-suggestion in such situations seems to be quite imperceptible. Jones (E.), " The Nature of Auto-Suggestion ", *The International Journal of Psa.*, vol. IV, pp. 3°4-5.

[2] Bradbury (M. K.),, " The Logic of the Unconscious Mind ", book review by J. C. Flügel, *The International Journal of Psa.*, vol. II, 1921, p. 128.

The marvellous plays a great part in all suggestion. It plays no less a part in leading the public to accept some of the extravagant claims put forward on behalf of suggestive and especially auto-suggestive therapy.

Auto-Suggestion

Even so anti-Freudian a psychologist as Watson recognizes the rôle of the father as the giver of suggestions, as healer and religious leader.[1] The psycho-analysts push this point further, and claim that the *imago* of a (hetero- or homo-) sexually attractive parent stands behind *all* suggestive phenomena.[2] Nor does the sharp distinction usually made between hetero- and auto-suggestion have validity.[3]

[1] " The chief medicine man of the family group is of course always the father. In the still larger group God or Jehovah takes the place of the family father. Thus even the modern child from the beginning is confronted by the dicta—be that his father, the soothsayer of the village, the God or Jehovah. Having been brought up in this attitude of authority, he never questions their written or spoken statements. He accepts them at their face value. He has never deviated from them, neither have his associates, and hence has never had an opportunity to prove or doubt their worth. This accounts for the hold religion and superstition have upon our life." Watson (J. B.), " Behaviourism ", *Psyche* (London, July, 1924).

[2] " We may therefore conclude that the characteristic of suggestion lies in the free development of the affects of communicated ideas, the forces usually hindering this development being neutralized by the presence of the *rapport* or concentration on the idea of the operator. It is generally agreed that this *rapport* consists of an emotional bond ; as is well known, psycho-analysts consider the bond to be sexual in nature and due to the re-animation of an infantile attachment to a parent." Jones (E.), " The Nature of Auto-Suggestion ", *The International Journal of Psa.* (London, 1923)', vol. IV, p. 297.

[3] " Indeed, Abraham points out that these hysterical states may either occur spontaneously or be induced through the presence of some person by whom the subject feels himself to be ' hypnotised '. Two features therefore stand out here ; the importance of auto-erotism, and of incestuous attachment to the father. We also note once again the great difficulty of distinguishing between hetero- and auto-suggestion, and this must incline us to the conclusion that either there is only one process concerned in all the phenomena grouped under these two names or else, if there are two, they must be extremely closely related." Jones (E.), " The Nature of Auto-Suggestion ", *The International Journal of Psa.* (London, 1923), vol. IV, p. 302.

Q

Thus Ernest Jones relates how :

" Some years ago I had the good fortune to treat a patient, who graduated highly in the Yoga Hierarchy. In the psycho-analysis of his case, which I published at length,[1] two features were specially prominent in this connection, and these were the same two as we noted in respect of the hysterical dream states. The part played by the idea of God-Father in the autohypnotic state was unmistakable."

Jones believes this to hold true generally, that the " self " which gives the auto-suggestion, is really modelled upon a memory of the father.

For one thing, religious self-absorption is closely connected with concentration on the thought of God. Again, the outer manifestations of the two kinds of suggestion are similar.[2]

In explanation Jones points out how :

" The energy that gives the ego-ideal its significance is wholly derived ultimately from narcissistic libido. There are three routes for this : (1) Directly from the original narcissism of the primary ego . . . ; (2) via the attachment to the father-ideal . . . ; (3) via the regression to narcissistic identification with the father that often takes place after a disappointment at the lack of gratification of object love."[3]

---

[1] *Jahrbuch der Psychoanalyse*, 1921, band. IV, p. 564.

[2] " Even in the case of religious trances we have noted the interrelation between intense self-absorption on the one hand, and concentration on the idea of an external person on the other. Then again, the actual manifestations of the two conditions are quite identical. They may be said to include all the effects that mental functioning can potentially bring about in both mental and physical fields, from the most complete delusional and hallucinatory formations in the former to the gravest interference with all kinds of bodily functions in the latter, and in rare cases even with life itself." Jones (E.), " The Nature of Auto-Suggestion ", *The International Journal of Psa.* (London, 1923), vol. IV, p. 305.

[3] *Idem*, p. 306.

Jones summarises his conclusions as follows :—

" Suggestion is essentially a libidinal process ; through the unification of the various forms and derivatives of narcissism the criticising faculty of the ego-ideal is suspended, so that ego-syntonic ideas are able to follow unchecked the pleasure-pain principal in accordance with the primitive belief in the omnipotence of thought. Such ideas may develop to their logical goal (beliefs, judgments, etc.), or regress to their sensorial elements (hallucinary gratification). The essential

We shall now proceed to the application of these principles in the various types of movements which we are studying.

ECONOMICO-POLITICAL TYPE

We are tied to the ways and beliefs of our fathers, not only by sentiments of loyalty to them, but also by the sense of authority which long habits of trustful obedience have developed in us. Thus, " X——— " feels that any question of the rightness of the institution of private property is settled when we find a definite pronouncement on the subject by the fathers. Rights are not derived, he says, from the consent of the sons to the arrangement. They go back to an earlier source which it is sacrilegious to question, and which is connected with the origin :

> " There have been many . . . formations of under-lying American principles. Perhaps none is better . . . than that . . . of the State of Ohio, which reads :
> " ' All men . . . have certain inalienable rights, which are those of . . . acquiring, possessing, and protecting property, and seeking safety.'
> " These rights are not derived from the consent of society and are not the grant of any government. They are natural and inalienable. Their roots are to be found in human personality."[1]

Wherever the point of departure is a religious one, there, naturally, the argument from authority is much

part of the unification in question is that between the real ego and the ego-ideal. The condition under which it takes place is that the repressed allo-erotic impulses are to be renounced. This is made possible by a regression of their libido in the direction of auto-erotism, which results in a further reinforcement of the narcissism. If the primary narcissism has been released and re-animated directly by concentration upon the ideal self, the process may be termed auto-suggestion. If it has been preceded by a stage in which the ego ideal is resolved into the earlier father-ideal, the process may be termed hetero-suggestion." Jones (E.), in *The International Journal of Psycho-Analysis* (London, 1923), vol. IV., p. 308.

[1] " X——."

in vogue. Thus, one writer says that no obedient son (Christian) who takes the father's commands as authority for what is right, can be a socialist (meaning communist ?) :

> "No Christian who accepts the Commandments as the basis of moral law can possibly deny the right of private individual property, seeing that this right is clearly recognised by the 8th and 10th Commandments.
> "If the Christian socialist admits this, he is clearly no socialist, if on the other hand he denies it he is clearly no Christian."[1]

HUMANITARIAN TYPE

I shall give an illustration of the working of some of these principles in the actual case of Kenyon and then generalize on their operation in the case of war-time psychology.

Kenyon

Some further facts in the history of Kenyon will tend to show the lasting effects upon his philosophy of certain suggestions from his father, manifested merely as slight signs of pride and approval. It was perhaps largely the very fact of his father generally interfering so much less in the boy's affair than the latter desired, which made him so responsive to the rare signs of paternal interest.

Kenyon's constructive activities seem always to have been a source of satisfaction to his father—perhaps they gratified vicariously some impulse of his own (he was very skilled with tools). At the age of seven, on one occasion, when Kenyon had built himself a boat big enough to get into, out of old sheet iron, the boy's skill was warmly commented on, in his hearing, by his

[1] "X——."

father. In later years, his skill in designing remained one of the few things his father openly praised.[1]

The results of the foregoing were seen in two directions. First : In a general way utilitarianism was stressed as against mere amusement *per se*. As early as he can remember, the boy resented the word " play " being applied to any of his occupations. He would answer with some heat : " I never play. I work ". In this he felt his father's approval. The excess of this attitude was bad inasmuch as it tended to cramp one side of his development. Games are even to-day distasteful to him : he takes lessons in them and manages to play them only by looking on them as a discipline.

Second : On the other hand, the resultant elimination of all frivolous activities has meant that a great deal has been accomplished in certain narrow channels, notably intellectual. The fact that Kenyon never read novels save as he was required to at school, was a matter of much pride to his father.

One effect which the whole thing had was that it biased him toward the school of utilitarian philosophy with all its humanitarian implications. He embraced this wholeheartedly from his first reading of J. S. Mill at the age of 16.

[1] Compare the effect of a similar attitude upon Marie Stopes, the birth-control leader (unfortunately for the purposes of this thesis she does not come under the designation of a son, but it is apparent from Maude's biography of Marie Stopes that she had many boyish traits) : " As a young girl, I met so many of my parent's friends, mostly people who were doing something in the world of thought, that it is difficult to say who influenced me, and who did not, but I clearly remember an outstanding influence from one talk with Sir Francis Galton and also from Mrs Alec Tweedy. . . . Once at a party at Robert Mond's country house, she introduced me to him as ' a girl who is going to do great things '. I felt it was incumbent upon me to live up to such an introduction." Maude (A.), *Life of Marie C. Stopes* (London, 1924), p. 24.

On another occasion :—" The continuous unconscious education which companionship with her father gave Marie, was supplemented by really expert lessons in carpentry. Her father always anxious she should not do things in a ' lady-like ' way, taught the girl . . . and both girls helped their father to put up many shelves and make arrangements for his specimens. This resulted in a passion to do things for herself." Maude (A.), *Life of Marie C. Stopes* (London, 1924), p. 30.

Kenyon carried his utilitarianism to its extreme implications. Even in the case of the few pure amusements which he enjoyed, he felt that a burden of proof rested upon their advocates to show that these increased the ultimate total of human happiness. He must be satisfied that they did not merely give present pleasure at the expense of making the individual more pleasure-loving so that he would in future be increasingly dependent on being so amused. Music and all art were called upon to justify themselves before a sceptical judge. I am struck by the identity of his attitude here with that expressed by the socialist writer, Upton Sinclair, who anathematizes :

" The lie . . . that art has nothing to do with moral questions . . . All art deals with moral questions, since there are no other questions.
" The lie that the purpose of art is entertainment and diversion, an escape from reality . . . this lie is a product of mental inferiority, and . . . the true purpose of art is to alter reality."[1]

The obverse side of this minimization of the importance of pleasures was that Kenyon greatly stressed the duty of creating favourable conditions for the happiness of others. He became for a time a vegetarian, and always afterwards was very moderate in the consumption of foods or the use of materials (fur, leather, etc.) which involved animal suffering. He gave assistance to various humanitarian movements, and to those which, like socialism or birth control, aimed at relief of the conditions of the masses. In particular, he was, during the war, an ardent pacifist.

Such a working out of the effects of encouragement from the father are, however, not the rule. The true father-loving type is oftener an authoritarian. Northumberland, whom we have already had occasion to cite on account of his father-orientation in the political and, incidentally, in the religious, arena is of opinion that :

[1] Sinclair (U.), *Mammonart* (Pasadena, 1925), p. 9.

" In the final resort, civilization must rest upon some principle of authority. Christianity has invested all legal authority with a religious sanction. When this motive fails to satisfy, society still possesses a bond of unity in national sentiment. Pure democracy repudiates nationality, and thus strikes at the root of every ideal on which our civilization has been based . . .

" There is no higher mission before any man to-day than that of fighting this movement in all those forms in which it may display itself."

This typical attitude of the authoritarian against democracy will generally be found to hold good against the run of humanitarian movements and especially against pacifism, which seems generally a defiance of the government.

War-time Psychology

When war is declared, the great majority of people who called themselves pacifists suddenly, but generally quite sincerely, decide to conform to the action of the majority. They accept the suggestions which fill the daily Press, regarding the enemy's villainy and our own altruism. They are overawed by the authority of rulers and officials into more or less enthusiastic decision that the thing to do now is to fight. No doubt a variety of motives, such as that of rescuing the mother-country and punishing the enemy-fathers, anticipating sadistically the infliction of suffering, finding in national glory a narcissistic self-expansion, or enjoying homosexually the being massed together with great numbers of other men, prepare the individual to receive war-like suggestions favourably. But the spark which touches off this magazine is often supplied by the actions of revered father-figures.

At such a time the various conservative institutions generally act together, and so are able to crush easily the comparatively feeble revolutionary elements such as the communists, socialists, the less respectable among the pacifist organizations, etc., which dare keep their colours flying.

The authoritative churches[1] (as opposed to a scattering of heretical sects) are, as we have said, always among the first to aid the recruiting sergeant and to fan, from their pulpits, the flames of hate. During the Great War, the Kaiser found in this quarter one of his strongest sources of moral support, much to the scandal of the *entente* peoples, who were counter-praying and counter-sermonising vigorously. A sample of the bellicose propagandist ammunition to be found in the authoritative word of the Heavenly father is approvingly cited by Hudson Maxim :

> " Let us quote again from the Scriptures :
> ' The Lord is a man of war '. (Ex. xv. 3).
> ' The Lord of Hosts is His name '. (Isa. li. 15).
> ' Blessed be the Lord my strength, which teacheth my hands to war, and my fingers to fight '. (Psa. cxliv, 1).

> " It is evident that the modern Christian misunderstands Christ's true mission, for he said :

> ' Think not I am come to send peace on earth ; I came not to send peace, but a sword '. (Matt. x. 34).
> ' I am come to send fire on the earth ' (Luke xxii. 49).
> ' And he that hath no sword, let him sell his garment and buy one . . . ' (Luke xxii. 36)."[2]

But this brings us directly to the next division of our chapter and the topic of authority in religion.

THE RELIGIO-THERAPEUTIC TYPE

The rôle played by the father in the formation of the boy's *super ego* is recognized by every mother when she

---

[1] But some of course more so, some less. In America the Roman Catholic and the Methodist churches were perhaps more passive than other large denominations during the war.

[2] Maxim (Hudson), *Defenceless America* (London, New York and Toronto), p. 51.

chides her little son : "Look at your daddy. He does (not do) so and so." This is the sense of Pythagoras' admonition to his followers to be seen but not heard, when he bids them :

"Govern your tongue above all things, following the gods " (fathers.)[1]

The authority of the fathers was the very basis of the conduct of the Therapeutæ.[2]

In like manner the Essenes, also, guided their conduct by the word of the fathers, and based on that authority their peculiar herbal therapy.[3]

It was perhaps chiefly to the Essenes, and also to the Therapeutæ, that St Augustine referred, when he admitted that

"That which is called the Christian religion existed among the Ancients."[4]

[1] Iamblicus, *Pythagorean Symbols With Explanations*, p. 75.

[2] " Each hut has a sacred chamber reserved for their sacred books, the Law, the Prophets, the Psalms, and other writings, ' by means of which religion and sound knowledge grow together into a perfect whole '.

" After praying at dawn, they devote the day to meditation upon the scriptures ; these include writings or commentaries ' drawn up by the ancient founders of their sect ' by which Philo probably means the literature current under the names of men like Enoch and Abraham, whom he regarded as the primeval ascetics and recluses, the ideal progenitors of the Therapeutic movement. The method of study is allegorical interpretation, and the outcome of it is the composition of sacred hyms. Prayers at sunset close the day. Such is the life in each hut. On the seventh day the various members meet for common worship ; they arrange themselves according to age, sitting on the ground with ' the right hand between the chest and the chin, but the left hand tucked down along the flank. The senior recluse then delivers an address, to which all listen in silence, merely nodding assent '." Philo, *De Vita Contemplativa*, as quoted by Moffatt (J.), in art. " Therapeutæ " in *Encyclopædia of Religion and Ethics*.

[3] " They display an extraordinary interest in the writings of the ancients, singling out in particular those which make for the welfare of soul and body ; through these they make investigations into the medicinal roots and the properties of stones, useful in the treatment of diseases." *Selections from Josephus*, transl. Thackery.

[4] " and never did not exist, from the beginning of the human race until Christ came in the flesh, at which time the true religion which already existed began to be called Christianity." St. Augustine, quoted by Urwick (E. J.), *Message of Plato* (London, 1920), p. lv.

Many of the old traditions of Egypt, therefore, even as they were introduced into Greece by Pythagoras, were passed on to Mohammedanism or to Christianity through the Therapeutæ and Essenes. We find them among the Dervishes and some Christian cults.

Dervishes

The influence of the authority of the priest-fathers and of the Koran (word of the Heavenly Father and of his prophet, Father Mohammed) and of various forms of suggestion is clearly brought out in Macdonald's description of the Dervish ceremony he attended in Cairo :

> " There was in it none of the irregulated transports, outbreaks, shriekings, which so often appear in what we call times of revival. The whole performance was kept carefully in hand. It was plain to me that throughout it all the Sheik who was presiding or his assistant—as it lasted a long time he was once or twice relieved by an assistant—one or other had his hand upon this great machine, was keeping in touch with it, holding it in and down.
> "Exactly as a conductor will regulate and keep hold of his orchestra ; so he played upon them, so he kept them within bounds. There was nothing there of the nature of an outbreak, nothing of the disgraceful scenes—if I may say it—which happen at revivals."[1]

I found an equally authoritative atmosphere at the Fontainbleau institute. Quite in keeping with the Mohammedan (Sufi) origin of many of Gurdiev's ideas, and with the atmosphere created by the divans, hangings and wealth of Persian rugs which adorn the pavilion, was the despotic character of Gurdiev's control. Although there was in nothing any compulsion based on fear of punishment, yet his word in all things was law.[2]

---

[1] Macdonald (D. B.), *Aspects of Islam*, pp. 164-6.
[2] We understand also that through his chief assistants he keeps himself minutely informed of the doings of each follower. Such centralized authority and such espionage, if foisted upon society at large, would represent a loss to mankind of the fruits of centuries of political struggle. Whether to accustom the students at the Institution to

Christian Cults

In Christendom, from time to time, some new sect has formed around the person of a prophet who revived this ancient tradition of healing illness by the authority of sacred paternal texts, and of such was Quimby :

> " Mr Quimby, although not belonging to any church or sect, had a deeply religious nature, holding firmly to God as the first cause . . . Mr Quimby was a great reader of the Bible, but put a construction upon it thoroughly in harmony with his train of thought."[1]

He presently ceased to call his method (which was the basis of Christian Science and of New Thought) hypnotic, as he had done in former times.   Yet it will be apparent that it had really not changed his technique greatly save that the authoritative suggestions were given now in the waking instead of in the trance condition.   But, as the present writer (among others) found in an experimental study of the two types,[2] there is absolutely no sharp demarcation, nor any distinction which is of kind and not merely of degree, between hypnotic and waking suggestion.   Quimby gives the following example of his technique :

> " When sitting by a sick person who had a pain in the left side, which I felt and described, I said, ' You think you have consumption '. The patient acknowledged it, saying that her physician had examined her lungs, and found the left one very much effected . . . I told her that her disease was in her mind."[3]

them may not be a social danger, is a question.   But for the successful working of Gurdiev's system for the correction of character-traits in his students, there are advantages in this method.   He must be the sole person to assign tasks, on the theory that very few men approach him in knowledge of how to do so to the best advantage of the individual concerned.   And for him to work with insight, obviously he must be accurately informed as to how each student is reacting to his regime.

[1] Quimby (Geo. A.), in *New England Magazine*, March, 1888.   Quoted by Dresser (A. G.), *Philosophy of P. P. Quimby*, p. 20.

[2] Hopkins (P.), *A Study of Motivation*, thesis submitted in partial fulfillment of the requirement for M.A. degree, Columbia University, New York, 1910.

[3] Quimby (P. P.), article partly quoted by Dresser (A. G.), *Philosophy of P. P. Quimby* (Boston, 1895), p. 62.

The popular movement embodying Quimby's ideas and known as New Thought had so great a vogue that its exponent, R. W. Trine, felt justified in writing a phrase which reveals the exaggerated importance which his movement attaches to herd action. As suggestion itself, on which they so much rely, is generally most conspicuous as a herd phenomena, it is only logical for the proponent of suggestion to welcome—and to exaggerate—the power of the herd mind :

> "Doctors are now compelled . . . into . . . mental therapeutics. There is no time for . . . scepticism or doubt or hesitation. He who lingers is lost, for the entire race is enlisted in the movement."[1]

A writer approvingly quoted by Marden on behalf of New Thought goes so far in the worship of herd-mindedness that he would submit all school children to the authority of paternal regulation as to what are " right thoughts " or " wrong ones " for them to hold. The extraordinary thing, however, is the defence rationalized on behalf of such a procedure, namely, that when all the " wrong ones " have been ruthlessly repressed (" expelled ") there will thereafter be " nothing to repress "—all being hidden, there will be " nothing to hide ".

> " The child taught to hold right thoughts and to expel wrong ones by governing its own mental realm . . . will grow up pure minded and truthful because of having nothing to hide, nothing to repress."[2]

If such is the close mental atmosphere in which the apostles of suggestive therapy would bring up the younger generation, we must not be greatly surprised if reverence for the father leads them to put up with a somewhat similar physical atmosphere.

> " We were the first to reach the little cottage . . . where M Coué usually sees his patients . . . Ventilation is a

[1] Trine (R. W.), *In Tune with the Infinite* (London, 1923), p. 37.
[2] Carter (M. E.), as quoted by Marden (O. S.), in *Every Man a King*, p. 8.

difficulty . . . to avoid a draught . . . the window is relentlessly shut. M Coué himself is, of course, thanks to self mastery, almost indifferent to any atmosphere, stifling or otherwise . . . The rest of us try to follow in his steps, and some of us are actually surprised at our success in not minding very much the airlessness of the room ; we have said to ourselves, ' This is doing me good '."[1]

But it is time now to bring to an end this, the last chapter of our thesis. It has brought to our attention some rather striking laudations of the principle of authority from an exponent of democracy and decrier of socialism. The same awe of the father was seen to move one individual toward utilitarianism, and another towards conservation of established values in civilization, and others to acquiesce in war. Naturally it played a tremendous part in religions, from the most ancient of them down to suggestive therapeutic cults of the present day.

This concludes the main body of my thesis. But I append below a Synopsis which is intended to help the reader to pass in review all the diverse material which has been herein presented, see it more as a whole, and weigh its value.

---

[1] MacNaughten (Hugh), *Emile Coué* (London, 1922), pp. 1-2.

SYNOPSIS

SYNOPSIS OF THE FOREGOING

WE have been drawing our own deductions in each chapter and section of this thesis, as we went along. So here I shall endeavour merely to pull these various strands together by way of rounding off and concluding this work.

Our Introductory Chapter, and the Introductory Remarks which headed the other chapters, had no purpose save to expound certain leading psycho-analytic ideas, the fruits of the researches of investigators. The need of brevity requires me to omit these from my summary, and review here only a part of the material which I myself have collected, and that chiefly by just giving heads of topics.

I will begin with the " Economico-Political " section of the Rescue Phantasy Chapter in Part One. Here we heard the rebel novelist Ibanez, after denouncing his king as tyrant, call his country a lady in a tower awaiting her rescuer (p. 6). The romantic strain was uppermost in Marx (p. 7) and Hyndman. Communism had a history confused with that of innovations in marriage, or rescue from the father (p. 8) and socialism aspired to rescue unfortunate womankind from prostitution (p. 9).

The " Humanitarian " section of this chapter represented Eder's picture of the Earl of Shaftesbury moved to works of mercy because a servant had been to him as a mother (p. 12).

In the " Religio-Therapeutic " section : We saw Quimby's phantasy of himself as Moses rescuing patients

241   R

from the Red Sea of medical beliefs and from doctors' semen-like ideas (p. 16). Mrs. Eddy and Dr. Coué endorsed pre-natal influence (p. 17). Nash broke with Adventist beliefs and the Elders who damned a motherly woman (pp. 17-18).

The second chapter dealt with the father as oppressor, etc.

In the "Economico-Political" section : we noted how Marx had broken his father's heart (p. 23), quarrelled with governments (p. 24), with most men friends (p. 25), and with the father-like Bourgeoisie (p. 25). Kenyon gave us a parallel for the people led astray by "professional economist" fathers (pp. 26-27). Hyndman, rejected by Marx because of the book (p. 27) or hat (p. 28) episode, wished to be self-created without a father (p. 28). The gulf between social classes lay partly in Marx' and Lenin's domestic pasts (p. 29). Marx' internationalism made him appear a father (p. 30) ; Flint and Asquith saw paternal tyranny in socialism (pp. 30-31). Russia and New York tried to be egalitarian in dress (pp. 31-32). Competition was a father-figure to socialists (p. 33), and protectionists (p. 33). Humbolt, Stirner, Paine, Shelley, and Emerson feared the paternal State (p. 34). Revenge was meted to the Pharoahs (p. 36), and democracy turned its father-leaders out (p. 36).

In the "humanitarian" section : We unearthed Bentham's resentment against his father (pp. 38-39). A journalist described the revolt of the Orient against English-speaking father-types (pp. 41-42). The United States was becoming hated as the world's banker-father (p. 43). Philpott's poem "War" called the father's penis "blood-rusted" (p. 43). Socialists and pacifists had a common enemy in fathers (p. 45). To the Molokan, an officer was a father (p. 46). War restrictions were resented as castration by the father (p. 47).

In the "Religio-Therapeutic" section : Free Thought was uncastrated potency (p. 48). Quimby, true founder of Christian Science (p. 49), opposed sowing semen-like thought-seeds (p. 49). Mrs. Eddy opposed parental intercourse (pp. 50-51), and felt as a son (pp. 51-52) to her bigoted father, and the doctor-fathers who could not aid her in her neurotic youth (p. 54). Quimby despised slaves to the doctors (pp. 55-56); Hardy called the father imbecile (p. 57).

Chapter III was on the father as monopolist and capitalist.

In the " Economico-Political " section : Burns and Quelch opposed the paternal virtues of thrift and industry (p. 61). Was immorality due to fathers or sons ? (p. 62). If altruism was father-like, some sons preferred egoism (pp. 62-63).

In the " Religio-Therapeutic section : The early Christians were communist-brothers (pp. 63-64). The papal father betrayed the rebel, Francis (pp. 64-65). Whoso obeyed the father in heaven would obey an industrial boss (p. 65). Hyndman resented his paternal inheritance being willed to religious, charities (p. 66). The churches were on the side of paternal privilege (p. 66).

Chapter IV was on " The Castrating and Killing Phantasies."

In the " Economico-Political " section : Paternal restrictions on teaching in the United States (pp. 78-79) and Comstock's distinction between fathers' liberty and sons' licence (p. 80), were combated by the Civil Liberties Union (p. 80). Catastrophic revolutionists sought to castrate the old father-controlled order (p. 85). Some sons boasted that castration was not permanent (pp. 83-84).

In the " Humanitarian " section : Criminals defied the father-symbolizing state (p. 86), hence many sympathised with criminals (p. 87). But criminals were also fathers (p. 87). To stop war, castrate the fathers by cutting off their property (p. 88).

In the " Religio-Therapeutic " section : Atheism banished father as prototype (p. 90). Bentham (p. 90),

Marx, Morris and Hyndman (pp. 91-92) were illustrative cases. Hyndman seldom mentioned his father
(p. 93). Baudoin, as a boy, wove death-phantasies
about his parents (p. 94).

Chapter V dealt with " Ambivalence " and the " God-
complex ".

In the " Economico-Political " section : Hyndman
thought co-operatives bourgeois (p. 98), and these
quarrelled with Unions (p. 99), yet capitalist-fathers
persecuted them (p. 99). Lenin became the father of
the " red " regime (p. 99), and communists paternally
disallowed free speech (p. 100). Labour's attitude to
them was self-thwarting (pp. 102-103). Before his conversion Spencer called socialism paternal slavery (p. 104).
Intolerance and venom betrayed Marx' god-complex
(p. 105). Schroeder described democratic anti-father
fictions (pp. 106-107).

In the " Religio-Therapeutic " section : Quimby read
the book of disease (p. 107) because of his wisdom, which
was God or Christ-father (p. 108), so he was omnipotent
over disease (p. 109). Mrs. Eddy was superior to talk of
anatomy (p. 109), since matter is unreal (p. 110). She
queened it while her hostesses drudged (p. 112), and her
word was equal to that of father-God (p. 110). Trine's
god-man was unlimited (p. 111). Marden's coming man
should be a king (p. 114). Pre-natal influence was
indorsed by Mrs. Eddy and Coué, who reduced all
problems of medicine and sociology to that of holding
correct opinions (p. 116). The father of Mazdazan
assumed fantastic titles (p. 117).

In Part Two of the thesis the first chapter was
on Anxiety, Conscience, Sense of Sin, and Self-
punishing.

In the " Economico-Political " section : Blatchford
humbly denied a son's right to himself (p. 131), and
the Fabians denied him choice of vocation (p. 131).
" X——" exonerated Father Civilization, blaming
human nature (p. 131). Kenyon could not be adult

nor fully join movements scorned by his father
(p. 132).

In the " Religio-Therapeutic " section : Comstock
found the father's word the only restraint to vice (p. 134).
Quimby equated filial reason to disease (p. 163), and
Coué despised mere theory (p. 135). Trine feared hatred
(p. 137). Marden's coming man would be without fear
(p. 138). The Essenes feared using father's name in an
oath (p. 138). Quimby equated error to matter or the
devil (p. 139) blamed not the father but the sons (p. 141)
and hoped to deduce a science (p. 141). So did Mrs
Eddy (p. 142), and Coué (p. 142). Trine rehabilitated
sorcery (p. 144). Self-punishment for sin against father
was practised by Dervishes (pp. 144-145), by the Gurdeiv
institute (p. 146) and by physical culturists (p. 147).

Chapter II dealt with persecution of the sons.

In the " Economico-Political " section : more sons
were political prisoners than ever before (p. 153). The
father-minded American Legion cowed a mayor
(pp. 153-154). Belloc wiped out successful rebel sons
with a stroke of his pen (p. 155).

In the " Humanitarian " section : Government officials
were class-conscious (p. 158). Maxim, Nietzsche and the
father-minded belittled pity (p. 158). Old men stayed at
home and sent sons to the war (p. 159). Some fathers
opposed abolishing war (p. 160). Prisons served to vent
animosity on sons (p. 161) as did also naval flogging
(p. 161). Burning a woman alive and crushing a baby
saved the father-race's culture (pp. 163-164) further
protected by the Klu Klux Klan (pp. 164-165).

Chapter III was on Homosexuality, Identification,
etc.

In the " Economico-Political " section : " X——-"
thought the fathers would have been surprised at the
sons' irreverence (p. 171). We should learn to speak
with the father's voice (pp. 171-172).

In the " Religio-Therapeutic " section : Sons danced
to honour the father among the Egyptians, Hebrews,

Therapeutæ, Greeks and Essenes (pp. 173-175). The same motive was found in the Dervish dhikr (p. 174), as at Kairoan (p. 176), and was found in some catholic cathedrals (p. 179). Adventists had their "sterilized dancing" (p. 179). Mazdaznan followers attained union with the father in exercises of breathing (pp. 177-178), bowing the knee (p. 178) or adoration (p. 178). Dervishes received seed through a *silsila* from the father (p. 180). In Quimby, father—wisdom—self (p. 181). Mrs. Eddy was the equivalent of father-Jesus (p. 181). Marden's coming man would experience one-ness with the blessed father (p. 181). Coué took Liebault as his father-type (p. 182).

Chapter IV was on Providence.

In the "Economico-Political" section : Hyndman was trustingly blind to "dark asian strands" (p. 187). Trust in father was unsuited to democracy (p. 188), but opened the way for the "strong man" (p. 189).

In the "Humanitarian" section : Block and Jordan prophesied that the fathers would not permit a war (p. 189). Ruskin derived all good from Father Mars (p 190).

In the "Religio-Therapeutic" section : Comstock protested against destroying the sense that father will do everything for us (p. 191). Mrs Eddy prescribed knowledge of the father as relief (p. 192). Trine based unlimited optimism on God (p. 192), to ask of whom is the way to get anything (p. 193). Dresser was an optimist because a loving father existed (p. 194). Marden derived a law of opulence from the Creator's plan (pp. 195-196). Coué's paternal words covered everything (pp. 196-197).

Chapter V treated of Loyalty.

In the "Economico-Political" section : The loyalty to Father Marx, Eder found, gave the Russian revolution stability (p. 199). On socialism and father-like superiority, Le Bon (p. 200) and Shaw (p. 200) disagreed. American revolutionaries had become fathers (p. 200) whose word was sacred (p. 201) but whom socialists called crooks (p. 201). The Fabians' irreverence shocked Hyndman (p. 203), who had adopted Marx' ideal father-land (p. 204) ; they would starve virtues (p. 206). Moscow committed a blasphemy against father (p. 206). Father Capitalism had a social purpose (p. 207). Justice would fall with Father Royalty (p. 207). We were not to blame the individual, but his creator (p. 207). " X——" reversed this (p. 209). Pearson would avenge the paternal state (p. 210). Some Fabians opposed equal status of sons (p. 210). Free Trade would rob fathers of servants (p. 210). Police-fathers gave freedom (p. 210). The British Constitution was perfect (p. 211). Our institutions were best because settled by our fathers (p. 212).

In the " Humanitarian " section : Father-loyalty became patriotism (p. 213). Military expenditure was but a transfer (p. 214). Tolstoy learned pacifism from his father-replacing elder brother (p. 214).

In the " Religio-Therapeutic " section : Pythagoras bade honour the fathers and not disbelieve (pp. 214-215). The Essenes reverenced ancestral ethics (p. 215). Com-stock would have father-despising atheists humble (p. 216) but found them bigoted (p. 217). Quimby blamed disease upon the sons (p. 217). Mrs Eddy asked reverence for her book (p. 219) and equated Father-Christ with Truth (p. 219).

The Final Chapter, number VI, was on Authority, Suggestion, etc.

In the " Economico-Political " section : " X——" claimed that rights did not depend on the consent of the sons (p. 227), and that no one who accepted the father's commandment could be a socialist (p. 228).

In the " Humanitarian " section : Kenyon's utilitar-ianism was due to paternal influence (pp. 228-229). Northumberland stressed paternal authority in civil-ization (pp. 230-231). Pacifists were overwhelmed by impulse to conform (p. 231). Militarists quoted the heavenly father's authority (p. 232).

In the " Religio-Therapeutic " section : Pythagoras bade us imitate the silence of the heavenly father (p. 233). The Therapeutæ (p. 233) and the Essenes (p. 233) guided life by the word of the father. Macdonald found Dervish ceremonies well governed by the paternal Sheik (p. 234). Gurdiev exerted similar authority (p. 234). Trine announced that doctors were compelled into psychotherapy by herd-action (p. 236). Coué's follower-sons accepted bad ventilation as wholesome for them (pp. 236-237).

I am aware that some of the instances which I have cited in this thesis to illustrate the influence of unacknowledged motivations have been strained. The reader will ask why these cases could not have been accounted for on conscious rational grounds. But it is only when the affect connected with any conduct is out of proportion to the requirements of the situation, that one is justified in deducing the existence of non-rational motives.

I ask the reader to put down any such straining of points not (as has too often been done where such things have occurred) to the discredit of the psycho-analytic view point or technique, but to my own inexperience, as a newcomer in this vast and complex field. I rest my case on the hope that the amount of material here collected is sufficiently large so that among it all there will still be enough valid matter to convince the reader.

INDEX

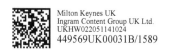